BE A \

BE A VEGETARIAN

Be a Part of Green Revolution

Edited by

ARUN JAIN

Publications

KALPAZ PUBLICATIONS

DELHI-110052

Be a Vegetarian

ISBN : 81-7835-346-6

Published in 2008 in India by
Kalpaz Publications
C-30, Satyawati Nagar, Delhi-110052
E-mail : kalpaz@hotmail.com
Phone : 9212729499

Laser Type Setting at : Master Computer's, Delhi
Printed at : Vishal Kaushik Printers, Delhi

DEDICATION

To my wife Simmi with whom I have matured over years and who has been there with me through thick and thin

Contents

Foreword

I have known the author for years and this book is written with conviction from a person who has followed vegetarianism both as legacy and choice.

I have read many a books and each of them has its own beauty. This book wonderfully sails through the historical aspect to the most modern development in the science of vegetarianism.

Readers are engaged in open and friendly discussion and are given honest answers.

Even though I too am a staunch vegetarian, it is beautiful to see how the reader is given a free choice and is rather persuaded than forced.

My suggestion to every reader would be to introspect after they have read the book and decide for themselves what's best.

I wish all the best to the author who is a close friend my mine and extend my wishes to every reader of this book.

Rajnath Singh

National President
Bhartiya Janta Party

Preface

With the first few steps in the 21st century, the world is realizing a new revolution. The old traditions are seen in new light; old practices are being revived in the light of new discoveries, new explanations and progressing science. Vegetarianism too fits into this category, the age old practice finding scientific support.

This book has been written in light of modern facts and researches done on vegetarianism at the same time, the religious aspect of vegetarianism has not been neglected and has been discussed in full details.

The book is not contempt of non-vegetarianism, as food is a matter of personal choice; however, it is a sincere effort to disclose and be an eye-opener to the truth behind non-vegetarianism and advocates vegetarianism emphatically. Vegetarianism has been presented not as a blind practice but with full scietific evidence in support of the food group choice.

Even if a single reader is persuaded towards vegetarianism or at least provoked to revise his/her dietary practices, the purpose of this book will meet its end.

Acknowledgements

This book has been an outcome of a long cherished desire of mine to spread words about vegetarianism.

In this effort there have been people known and unknown who have shaped my thought process knowingly and unknowingly. Not only would I acknowledge them but also my traditions and environment of upbringing with open-mindedness and in new lights of knowledge.

To name a few first of all I would thank my parents who made me what I am today, my wife Simmi who has been an inspiration and support throughout, without whom this book was an impossibility. Not to be forgotten my children- Devpriya who is more of a friend to me rather than daughter, Shivangi who has always insisted on the genuineness of the work and Shirish who helped me with his technical knowledge.

Last but not the least it will be a pleasure to acknowledge my friends and also Kalpaz Publications who have helped me with their expertise because of which the book has taken its final shape and is presented to the reader.

Arun Kumar Jain

1

Introduction

With the increase in the awareness and movement toward vegetarianism this book will take you on a journey into various aspects of vegetarianism.

Etymology

It is often claimed that the word "vegetarian" was invented with the formation of the first Vegetarian Society in 1847. In fact, their website claims "*[they] created the word vegetarian from the Latin 'vegetus' meaning 'lively' (which is how these early vegetarians claimed their diet made them feel) in 1847...*" and "*[the] term vegetarian has nothing to do with vegetables, but is taken from the Latin word for lively-vegetus.*"

Subdivisions of Vegetarianism

Vegetarianism has several subdivisions. Some of them of interest to our subject are:

(i) Lacto-ovo Vegetarians

(ii) Lacto Vegetarians

(iii) Ovo Vegetarians

(iv) Pollo Vegetarians

(v) Pesco Vegetarians

(vi) Vegans

Lacto-ovo *vegetarians* are those people who consume milk and eggs in addition to vegetables and fruits but don't consume meat of any kind. Such kind of vegetarians are considered to be practicing vegetarians in the western world where consumption of milk and eggs is an accepted practice amongst vegetarians. This, however, does not go down well with some Eastern countries where vegetarianism excluded consumption of eggs.

Lacto vegetarians are those people who consume milk and dairy products in addition to plant food. Such vegetarianism are common to India where milk is seen as an essential part of vegetarian diet. However, religious sentiments in India advocate that offspring of milk-giving animals are given a fair share before their milk is used for human consumption.

Ovo vegetarians are those who eat eggs but not meat.

Pollo vegetarians eat poultry products but not any other kind of meat.

Pesco vegetarians consume fish but refrain from taking any other kind of flesh.

We may exclude Pollo and Pesco Vegetarians from the class of vegetarians as they resort to eating of flesh. Lacto-ovo vegetarians and Ovo vegetarians can at best be described as semi-vegetarians. (Especially consumption of those eggs that have been fertilized)

There is another microscopic community of people who are vegetarians in the strict sense of term. They are called ***Vegans.*** They avoid taking all kinds of animal products such as milk, dairy products, honey etc. besides the meat. Such people suffer from some physical ailments on account of non-consumption of milk.

Other than Vegans, all over the world communities, milk is accepted as a vegetarians food. This is so because milk is not procured by killing of animals or putting them to any kind of torture. Most societies take care that the offsprings of milch animals do not suffer on account of human consumption of milk. They are offered a fair amount of suckling to meet their bodily needs. Alternative diets are also offered to them.

Encyclopaedia of Ethics defines vegetarianism as a diet of grains, vegetables, fruits, nuts and seeds, and dairy products and rejects dead animal bodies as a source of food.

Vegetarianism as a food practice goes down to our early ancestors. It may look surprising to note that our early ancestors lived for several million years on a vegetarian diet. Australian aborigines and Kung-san tribe of South Africa still live under conditions similar to those of our early mustangs. Studies on their food habits show that most of them live on a vegetarian diet. Fruits, seeds, nuts and vegetables are the staple foods of these groups. Contemporary studies on "hunter-gathers" suggest that early humans lived primarily on diet of plant foods. A portrayal of early humans as "gatherers" rather than 'hunters' is more accurate.

VEGETARIANISM THROUGH AGES

Our Earliest Ancestors

Our hominid ancestors evolved over a period of 24 million years and, according to Spencer (an English philosopher, (27 April 1820 - 8 December 1903)), for all but one-and-a-half million of these years lived on an almost completely vegetarian diet, except for occasional insects and grubs. Spencer suggests that lack of a varied plant and fruit diet may have been the reason Neanderthal man died out, while Cro-Magnon man, our direct ancestor, survived. The Cro-Magnons lived in a more temperate climate and had ready access to plentiful supplies of plants and fruit, while the Neanderthals, who lived in the icy wastes of northern Europe, were forced to subsist mainly on flesh food.

Greece

Vegetarianism, like other good ideas originated in ancient India in Asia, but in Europe it certainly originated in the ancient Greeks where Porphyry and Pythagoras were the best known practicing vegetarians.

Pythagoreans however did not publicize their vegetarianism for the fear of being enunciated as 'subversives' in a society that promoted gallant through killing of poor helpless and armless creatures. **Pythagoras** (*approx. 580-500 BC)* promoted and identified the health as well as spiritual benefits of vegetarianism. It was believed by Pythagoras and his followers that humans as well as have souls and that after death an animal may take rebirth as a human being and vice-versa, they believed in equality of souls. So they advocated that animals should not be killed and eaten.

Empedocles of Acragas *(c. 490-430 BCE)*, a pupil of Pythagoras suggested that all living things were on the same spiritual plane, indicating he was influenced by Pythagorean spirituality. Like Pythagoras, he believed in the transmigration of souls between humans and animals and followed a vegetarian lifestyle.

Socrates recommended a vegetarian diet because it would allow a country to make the most intelligent use of its agricultural resources. He warned that if people began eating animals, there would be need for more pasturing land. "And the country which was enough to support the original inhabitants will be too small now, and not enough."

The list of the other advocates of vegetarianism also includes Pluto, Plutarch, **Epicurus and Diogenes**. They favoured vegetarianism for a variety of reasons. In *'The*

Republic' **Pluto** suggests a vegetarian diet best suited for an ideal society of his imagination. Other Greek Philosophers and thinkers rejected eating animal flesh from aesthetic point of view.

Aristotle, pupil of Plato however believed differently and said that there is a hierarchy in nature and because plants are eaten by animals so they are superior and so is human to animals. his pupil **Theophrastus** (?372-?287BC) however began to work on his own Inquiry into Plants and Growth of Plants, and his own findings and thoughts differ from his teacher's in quite radical way. He did not think that animals existed for the sake of humans, and thought killing animals unnecessary and unjust, and that the habit of eating them must have begun when war destroyed crops. If plants and vegetable food were abundant there was no need to eat animal flesh.

Plutarch stated: "I am astonished to think what appetite first induced man to taste of a dead carcass or what motive could suggest the notion of nourishing himself with the flesh of animals which he saw, just before, bleating, bellowing, walking, and looking about them."

Rome

Many other ideas including vegetarianism were borrowed by the Romans from Greeks. Among those who championed the cause of vegetarianism in Rome are Seneca-the philosopher, and Ovid-the poet.

Seneca, the greatest of the Stoics wrote: "To abstain from the flesh of animals is to foster and to encourage innocence." In a later statement he claimed: "I resolved to abstain from flesh meat, and at the end of a year the habit of abstinence was not only easy but delightful."

Ovid, in the fifteenth book of his "Metamorphoses", puts into the mouth of Medea a forcible disquisition upon the

Golden Age: "Blest is the produce of the trees and in the herbs which the earth brings forth, and the human mouth was not polluted with blood."

Church

The utterly wrong idea that animals were on earth for the convenience and use of human beings spread among the Europeans, and which still prevails in their minds, with the spread of Christianity and the fall of Rome. Christian saints like Augustine and Thomes Aquinas provided intellectual rationalization for the exploitation, killing and eating of animal by humans. They argued that only humans have souls, rationality and free wills. This view in still accepted by majority of Christians.

The Heretics

Another big surge in vegetarianism came from the Manicheans in the early centuries AD. The Manicheans were a sect of "heretics" with vegetarianism as the centre of their beliefs, and were much reviled by the Christians. [It is for this reason that the book is called the Heretic's Feast] Manicheanism survived in the Near East as late as the seventh century AD and kept a foothold in China as late as the 16th century, the Manicheans being known as "vegetarian demon worshippers."

Renaissance

Renaissance brought about many changes in Europe in the field of classical art, philosophy and science. But to rediscover vegetarianism, the European took a little longer. During the early Renaissance period, an open vegetarian ideology was a rare phenomenon. Famine and disease were rife as crops failed and food was short. Meat was largely a scarce and expensive luxury for the rich. It was during this period that there was to be a rediscovery of ancient classical philosophy.

The famous genius and maestro Leonardo Da Vinci was a pioneer in being a confirmed vegetarian of his time. He writes:

"I have from an early age adjured the use of meat, and the time will come when men, such as I, will look upon the murder of animals as they now look upon the murder of men."

It was after advent of Charles Darwin's theory of evolution that a vegetarian "Renaissance" occurred in the West; this theory destroyed the notion that animals were fundamentally different from humans. Darwin challenged all sorts of justifications-religious or political-for killing and eating animals. His new view of animals as distant kin of humans made people thinks of animal rights-which is gaining strength these days-and people abstained from eating flesh. In the beginning they were said to be following the "Pythagorean diet."

Enlightenment

With the Enlightenment of the eighteenth century there emerged a new appraisal of man's place in the order of creation. Arguments that animals were intelligent feeling creatures were voiced and moral objections were raised as there was an increasing distaste for the mistreatment of animals. Amongst western religions there was a re-emergence of the view that, in fact, flesh consumption was an aberration from God's will and the genuine nature of humanity.

19th Century

It was the time that first written works by Europeans appeared on vegetarianism. Writers like P.B. Shelley and Jolstoy advocated for adopting vegetarianism as lifestyle resulting into formation of Christian groups working for the cause of vegetarianism. Shelly was fervent in his renunciation of meat consumption, convinced of the healthy advantages a meat-free diet could offer. Shelley also added a political dimension to the cause of vegetarianism by pointing out the inefficient use of resources. Meat was still at this time the habitual reserve of the privileged and Shelley cited meat production as a reason for food shortages among society's most needy.

Members of the "Bible CHRISTIAN Church" (1809) championed the cause of vegetarianism with a belief that Christ's teachings of mercy should be extended to animals, and that the Christians have a duty to do mercy to all creatures. Later the members of this group formed the first secular vegetarian organization in 1847 called "Vegetarian Society." They were the first to use the term 'Vegetarian' coined from Latin word 'Vegetus'-meaning fresh, lively, active or vigorous. Many members of the Society believed that salt and condiments were stimulants and as bad as alcohol. This led to vegetarian food being enormously bland. At this time, too, vegetarianism became equated with moral earnestness, do-good and the higher grounds of purity and moral rectitude. Meat was considered a generator of lust. Vegetarianism even went hand in hand with abstention from alcohol. Because British beef was regarded as one of the positive forces behind the growth of the British Empire, vegetarianism was very quickly relegated to the level of a joke by the rich and powerful.

20th Century

But time has its own twists. With the increasing tussle between vegetarianism and non-vegetarianism, finally vegetarianism managed to put a feet down post world war two when the economy of nations favored the cause of vegetarianism in their interest.

Later in the century environmental reasons of adopting vegetarianism, along with more healthy and natural lifestyle and more acceptance of eastern with the western culture have led more and more people to adopt vegetarianism. (However contrary is also to be noted where more and more westerners are adopting vegetarianism, more and more of previously predominantly vegetarian society of India is turning non-vegetarian as an influence from western society.)

Today various vegetarian societies around the world disseminates information on vegetarianism in the form of essays and lectures inspiring people to adopt Vegetarianism in order to form a more civilized society.

International Vegetarian Union

In the year 1908 the 'International Vegetarian Union' was formed with an aim to organize conferences at which vegetarians from around the world meet and share information. Even today, the union is active in this direction. Noble fellows like John Wesley—founder of Methodism, William Booth—founder of Salvation Army; Ellen Gould White—confounder of Seventh-day Adventists, G.B. Shaw-famous dramatist and Mahatma Mohan Das Karamchand Gandhi did everything to promote Vegetarianism; by all that these organization and personalities did was not sufficient.

A new wave of awareness, marking the role and importance of vegetarian diet in maintaining health—physical and mental both—came with new researches in the fields of nutrition and medical science, which brought major implications for the course of vegetarianism in the late 20th century. This awareness provided a broad pathway for new converts to the vegetarian cause.

The organizations and individuals who advocated the cause of vegetarianism, they saw many things behind it through their own perspectives—ethico-religious, aesthetic, scientific, economic health and nutrition.

Ethics and Vegetarianism

Ethics is a branch of philosophy defined as the "science of morals," while ethic is the "system of guiding principles." So, ethics can be said to be the mother of religion. Ethical dement of non-violence or non-killing runs through many of the great world religions arising from a variety of influences like asceticism, the belief in reincarnation; respect for all beings; the belief that eating animal flesh contributes to the degeneration of spirituality and finally non-violent ethics. Hinduism, Buddhism and Jainism all promulgate the theory of *Ahimsa*—non injury to sentient beings—and have strong vegetarian traditions. But Jainism requires it as a religious practice.

Christianity and Judaism hold that paradise was vegetarian (Genesis 1:29).

Apart from religious arguments ethical support for stricter vegetarian diets comes from animal rights and animal welfare arguments such as popularized by Peter Singer and John Regan. Many in the animal rights movements became vegetarians because they believed that it was inherently wrong to slaughter animals for food, no matter how humanely (?) they might have been killed.

The beginning of ethical vegetarianism is the knowledge that other creatures have feelings like that of humans. This knowledge encourages one to extend personal awareness to encompass the suffering of others; thus refuting the misconception of "humane slaughter of animals." Many people now days have been lulled into a sense of complacency thus presumably removing any possible humanitarian objection to the eating of animal flesh. Unfortunately, nothing could be further from the actual facts of life and death. The entire life of a captive 'food animal is an unnatural one of artificial breeding, vicious castration and hormone stimulation; feeding of an abnormal diet for fattening purposes and eventually long rides in intense discomfort to the ultimate end. Journal of the North American Vegetarian Society rejects the "humane slaughter of animals" in following word—" The holding pens, the electric prods and tail twisting, the object terror and fright, all these are still very much a part of the most 'modern' animal raising, shipping and slaughtering. To accept all this and only oppose the callous brutality of the last few seconds of the animal's life, is to distort the word 'humane.'"

The truth of animal slaughter is not at all pleasant—commercial slaughter houses are like visions of hell, even worse than that. Screaming animals are stunned by hammer blows, electric shock or concussion guns. They are hoisted into the air by their feet and moved through the factories of death on mechanized conveyor systems. Still alive, their throats are sliced and their flesh in cut off while they bleed to death. I am very much confident that many people would take up vegetarianism if they visited a slaughter house, or if they themselves had to kill the animals they ate. Such visits should be made compulsory for meat-eaters.

Plutarch challenged to the flesh-eaters, "If you declare that you are naturally designed for such a diet, than first kill for yourself what you want to eat. Do it, however only through your own resources, unaided by cleaver or cudgel or any kind of axe."

In an essay titled 'On Eating Flesh' he wrote," can you really ask what reason Pythagoras had for abstinence from flesh? For my part I wonder both by what accident and in what state of mind the first man touched his mouth to gore and brought his lips to the flesh of a dead creature, set forth tables of dead, stale bodies and ventured to call food and nourishment the pets that had a little before bellowed and cried, moved and lived. It is certainly not lions, nor wolves that we eat out of self-defense; on the contrary, we ignore these and slaughter harmless, tame creatures without stings on teeth to harm us. For the sake of a little flesh we deprive them of sun of light, of the duration of life they are entitled to by birth and being." He was inspired by the famous genius of geometry and mathematics Pythagoras who said, "Oh, my fellow men, do not defile your bodies with sinful foods. We have corn, we have apples, bending down the branches with their weight, and grapes swelling on the vines. There are sweet flavoured herbs and vegetables which can be cooked and softened over the fire, nor you are denied mild or thyme scented honey. The earth affords a lavish supply of riches of innocent foods, and offers you banquets that involve no bloodshed or slaughter, only beasts satisfy their hunger with flesh and not even all of those, because horses, cattle and sheep live on grass."

Alexander Pope expressed the opinion that: "Nothing can be more shocking and horrid than one of our kitchens sprinkled with blood and abounding with the cries of expiring victims or with the limbs of dead animals scattered or hung up here and there."

Leo Tolstoy wrote, "By killing animals for food man suppresses in himself, unnecessarily, the highest spiritual capacity—that of sympathy and pity toward living creatures like himself—and by violating his own feeling becomes cruel." He further warned," While our bodies are the living graves of murdered animals, how can we expect any ideal conditions on earth?"

The famous romantic poet P.B. Shelley was a committed vegetarian. In his essay 'A Vindication of Natural Diet' he observed, "Let the advocate of animal food force himself to a decisive experiment on its fitness, and as Plutarch recommends, tear a living lamb with his teeth and plunging his head into its vitals, stake his thirst with the steaming blood...., then, and only would he be content."

Sir Richard Phillips, who died in 1842 and was High Sheriff of the county of Middlesex, was an ardent vegetarian from the age of twelve when he visited a slaughterhouse. The philanthropist and prison reformer, John Howard, was a practicing vegetarian whose influence and concern affected many aspects of life in his own time and since. He claimed that his diet gave him immunity against "gaol fever" which was prevalent in the many filthy prisons he visited.

Leonardo Da Vinci wrote, "Truly man is the king of beasts, for his brutality exceeds theirs. We live by the death of others. We are burial places." He added hopefully, "The time will come when men will look upon the murder of animals as they now look upon the murder of men." Mahatma Gandhi felt that ethical principles are a stronger support for life long commitment to a vegetarian diet than reasons of health. "I do feel", he stated," that spiritual progress does demand at some stage that we should cease to kill our fellow creatures for the satisfaction of our bodily wants." He also said, "The greatness of a nation and its moral progress can be judged by the way its animals are treated."

Ellen White, founder of The Seventh Day, Adventists, says that the body is God's temple, and as such, should not be abused through the use of alcohol, tobacco, or meat. She also advocated the use of natural, unrefined foods. Today there are about two million Seventh-Day Adventists in the United States, and although it is not necessary to be a vegetarian to belong, about one half follow a lacto-ovo-vegetarian diet (a small proportion of them are vegan). Consistent with their emphasis on health, the Seventh-Day Adventists operate numerous clinics, sanitariums, and hospitals, as well as a medical school and research centre in Loma Linda, California. They also produce a variety of vegetarian foods for sale, specializing in products that simulate the texture and appearance of meat.

In 'Animal Liberation' and subsequent publications philosopher Peter Singer presented a utilitarian argument for vegetarianism based on the principle of equality of interests. He argued that the creatures with perceptions and the ability to feel pain should be afforded equality of interest with humans. Utilitarianism attempts to find a solution that allows the most favourable balance of pleasure and pain, i.e. good and bad. Considering that meat-eating is unnecessary for human health, the pleasure enjoyed by humans in trivial compared with the suffering inflicted on animals. Thus, the best balance of pleasure over suffering can be achieved through vegetarianism. Singer suggested, on this basis, humans should abstain from eating animal flesh (including fish), dairy products or eggs.

Further than Singer, goes John Regan is 'The Case for Animal Rights', arguing that animals have certain fundamental rights similar to those ascribed to humans. He is of the opinion that animals as well as humans are capable of acting autonomously, have preferences and posses ability to act to their will and to achieve their respective goals. He writes and I quote, "The principal right of all moral agents (animals and humans) is the right the respectful treatment. This includes the rights not to be killed (no matter how painlessly) because you cannot exercise your other rights if someone has deprived you of life."

Such arguments are enough to establish that no morally relevant differences exist between humans and the rest of the animal kingdom. But it is sad that differences do exist, however surprisingly difficult to demonstrate. With our increasing knowledge and understanding of animals, the continuities between humans and other animals appear to be stronger than earlier.

Religious Argument

All major religious scriptures enjoin man to live without killing unnecessarily, to have a feeling of fraternity towards all creatures of God, to have pity on weaker and to live in harmony with Nature. The Old Testament instructs, "Thou Shalt not kill." (Exodus 20:13). People often mistake this commandment as referring only to murder. The Buddhist sutras often mention the "power of mercy." The 'Sangam Sutra' says, "If we eat the flesh of living creatures, we are destroying the seeds of compassion." Absolute non-violence of thought and action in the very fundamental principle of the teachings of Jainism; and "*Ahimsa parmo dharma*," the Ved-sutra is the quintessence of Hinduism; Hindu scriptures consider every living being a part of God and lay utmost stress on '*Ahimsa*' (non-violence), compassion, love, forgiveness and such other virtues. All the Gurus of Sikhism have repeatedly, underlined the importance of non-violence and mercy, as has been said in the Adi Granth (p:1253) – "Himsa tou mante nahin Chooti, Jiya daya nahin pali." An Islamic authority Mr. Al-Hafiz B.A. Massi, in his book 'Islamic concern for Animals', has described all acts of torturing of animals as sin. He quotes Prophet Mohammed from *Quran* Mazid as under:

> "He who takes pity even on a sparrow and spares life, Allah will be merciful on him on the day of judgement."

Though mainstream Christianity never generated a strong tradition of Vegetarianism, in Genesis (1:29) we find God himself proclaiming, "Behold I have given you every herb-bearing tree, in which the fruit of the tree yielding seed, it unto you shall be for meat." And in later books of the Bible, Major Prophets condemn meat-eating. Majority of Christians believe that Christ ate meat and give references to meat in the New Testament. But a close study of the original Greek manuscripts shows that the vast majority of the words translated as "meat" simply mean "food" or "eating" in the broadest sense. For example, in the Gospel of St. Luke (8:55) we read that Jesus raised a woman from dead and "Commanded to give her meat." The original Greek word translated as 'meat' is 'phago' which means only 'to eat.' The Greek word for 'meat' is '*Kreas*', and this word has never been used in connection with Christ. Nowhere in the New Testament is there any direct reference to Jesus eating meat. This is in line with Isaiah's famous prophecy about Jesus's appearance, "Behold a virgin shall conceive and bear a son, and shall call him name Immanuel.

The Jewish Christians believed in simple living, pacifism and vegetarianism, for whom Jesus was a prophet loyal to the law and was a few. They opposed meat-eating and sacrifice of animals in the temple. There are frequent passages, in both Homilies and Recognitions, attacking animal sacrifice. Homilies state that God did not want animals killed at all (3.45) and condemns those who taste or eat meat at all (7.4, 7.8). This opposition to animal sacrifice and support of vegetarianism is one of the most distinctive features of Jewish Christianity mentioned by Epiphanies as well as in the Homilies and Recognitions.

Thus, all major religious forces direct humanity to be kind to animals and refrain from killing them.

These as well many other aspects of vegetarianism are detailed in the chapters to come.

2

Religion and Vegetarianism

Whole of this universe is run by a supreme authority which we call *God, Nature,* the *Creator* or give it any other name or form. Man has often tried to invade into the work of nature and undermine its authority but has always been convinced by the end results that the Creator is Supreme. Despite advancements in science and technology and man's untiring efforts, man has been unable to create man and depends upon nature for reproduction as he does for many other things.

This brings us to the fact that the universe is run by certain laws. These laws of the nature form the basis of religion which is nothing but a discipline born out of governing laws of nature and guides a man into a way of life.

Religion

Religion thus is a discipline in life. This is influenced by and is the outcome of the environmental needs of a particular region. Different regions of the world have seen rise of different religions on account of different types of environment settings there.

Religion has the single-most important influence on a man's life. A person may or may not be religious-minded, but all through out his life, his interaction with religion remains a regular fixture. All important occasions in a man's life have the bearing of religion on him from the time of birth till death occurs. A man might feel like to keep distance from religion but how can he escape from its influence with his parents, wife, kids, friends and all those in society with whom he interacts harping on religion and religious ceremonies. Or can he stop those loudspeakers, radio and TV broadcasts which preach religion. The phenomenon is not unique to a town, city or country but is universal in nature. When such is the influence of religion on life, can food, a source of life, remain aloof from it? Sure, our food consumption habits are greatly shaped by the religion we follow. Everyone is born a vegetarian but is later influenced by the prevailing food habit in family and society.

Food and Religion

All religions prohibit killing of harmless and innocent living beings. That should suffice to suggest that killing of animals for food is not approved by any religion. Somehow, some people argue that certain religions have no objection to meat-eating; this they do to satiate their appetites while maintaining their ethical standards. This is utterly untrue. Most religions have detailed the harmful impacts of meat-eating and called it the enemy of longevity and a source of degradation of man's body, soul and morals. That is to say that only a vegetarian diet is good for man's body as well as his soul. To take the argument further ahead, let us find out what various religions have to say on the issue of vegetarianism.

Hinduism

Of the four major religions, namely, the Hinduism, the Christianity, the Islam and the Buddhism, Hinduism is the oldest. Even other religions are of recent origin when compared to Hinduism. Since ancient times, Hinduism has promoted vegetarianism and highlighted meat as the food of *Rakshas* or the evil. The major Hindu scriptures that shape the opinion of the Hindus and influence their minds greatly are The *Vedas*, the *Mahabharta*, the *Ramayana* and the *Bhagwat Gita*. These holy scriptures stress on *Ahimsa*, compassion, love, forgiveness and such other virtues. Meat-eating has been described as totally sinful and leading to decline of soul. In or '*Anushasane Parva*' of the *Mahabharata*, Bhishma Pitamaha has described all those who eat meat, trade in meat and those who kill animals for their flesh as sinners. He opined that any one who eats meat of others in order to increase his own meat will never be able to live in peace in his next birth, whichever form he may take. Any living being that is slain claims, "Mas Bhakshyate Yasmad Bhakshishya Tamapapyaham" i.e. "Today he consumes me, some day I will eat him"

The Srimada Bhagwat Gita classifies food into three categories:

(i) *Satvik food* : Foods like fruits, vegetables, cereals, pulses, nuts, milk, butter, etc. which promote longevity, intellect and strength and provide pleasure, peace of mind, compassion, non-violence and equanimity and save the body, mind and heart from all impurities, fall under this category.

(ii) *Rajasik food* : Such foods include very hot, sour, bitter, spicy and dry substances. Such foods lead to perverted feelings, sorrow, disease and tensions.

(iii) *Tamsik food* : Stale, juiceless, half-cooked evil-smelling, rotting, impure, intoxicating materials, and meat, etc. are tamsik food. These foods prompt men to indulge in evil-deeds, cloud their intellect, give rise to disease, laziness and other evil qualities.

Doctrine of Rebirths

Doctrine of rebirths as set out in scriptures suggests that one attains the human form only after going through eighty-four lakh forms and cylces of birth and death. If this be so, all living beings are us through our earlier births. In such a case, if we consume meat, we are consuming the meat of one of our relatives.

Quoting Atharva Veda (8.6.23), "Ye Ammana Mas Madanti Paurnusheyam che ye Kavi Gaurhan Khadanti keshwastanto Nashyamasi."

i.e. Whoever eats raw or cooked flesh or whoever destroy a foetus shall be destroyed by us from here.

In *Satyartha Prakasha* Maharishi Dayanada suggests that by eating meat the temperament of a person is likely to become violence prone. Those who eat meat or consume liquor, their bodies and semen become contaminated.

According to the Hindu philosophy all living beings possess a soul. The soul is described by Krishna in the *Bhagawat Gita* as being the source of conscious and the active principle that activates the body of every living being. In the *Vedas* it is held that before evolving into the human form a soul is held in the lower species. Step by step it moves from a lower species to next higher species before ultimately residing in a human body. It is here in this form that soul turns its consciousness towards God and at the time of death it is transferred back to the spiritual world. The soul has thus to remain engaged in various forms for a preset duration and this duration must complete for the peaceful entry of the soul into the spiritual world. By killing of animals, the period of engagement of a soul is cut short and this creates an impediment to the orderly transition of the soul. This act implicates the killer and meat-eater as being sinners and must meet reaction for conducting a sinful activity.

Traditional Practice in a Hindu Family

Vegetarianism is traditionally practiced in orthodox Hindu families and children don't even know whether meat is also a variety of food till they learn through their own experiences. Dr. S. Jayaraman in a piece "The Day I Saw a Meat-Eater" in *Hinduism Today,* October 1994 recounts his childhood experience thus,

"Having been born in a south Indian orthodox family, I was never told that one could live on foods of animal origin during my school days in Madras. We had to carry our lunch packets for consumption during recess as there were no school canteens. I had no exposure to the sight of a person actually eating meat until I got out of school. Our parents and grand parents told us that we will be committing acts which will invite God's wrath if we have, let alone kill animals, for any reason except in self-defense. It deeply and unshakably, put it in our mind that any animal has the same right to live as we do. God had ordained that no animal can be harmed for pleasure, or on purpose, by us.

It was later when I entered the Madras veterinary college that I had the real exposure, not only to my friends' actually consuming meat but also to the science of raising animals and birds exclusively for satisfying the human palate and food needs. The subject of meat inspection was part of my curriculum. Necessarily any student of meat science had to handle meat, and in making the score card judgment of meat, he had also to taste meat and record his score. My schooldays and the unshakable faith and conviction imbibed in me due to the teachings of my parents, grand parents, uncles and aunts, prevented me from this unpleasant act. I was lucky in that some meat-eating classmates would always oblige me by tasting meat and giving the opinion which I would record as mine. With skill in this clandestine practice, acquired relentlessly in abundant measure, I could fudge my entry on this point even in the university examination, without any advance result. Believe it or not, I had this way carried on successfully, as a meat inspector in the earlier part of my service when I had to do meat inspection for three years. I also functioned quite successfully as the government of India's Licensing Authority under the Meat Food Products Order in 1973, without taking any meat what-so-ever. I have remained a vegetarian all along.

How Hinduism helps to create in young malleable minds the virtues of vegetarianism can be seen from the instance I cite below, which is on the far end of the other side of the scale. One day, in February, 1967, in Sydney, Australia, while I was walking to my college from home after the lunch break, I saw a tiny bird sitting on the pavement and chirping at the sun, I saw the bird suddenly collapse, but not die, following a gunshot sound. What I saw thereafter was a ghastly sight. A boy in his teens, toting a shotgun, walked towards the collapsed, gasping half alive bird, crushed it with his foot and dumped it in the roadside trash-bin.

As the logic of his action passed my comprehension, I asked him, "Why?" I was stunned by his reply, "I was practicing target shooting at tiny objects. "Could there be a more barbaric way of target practice? I thought. Even in the wildest of dreams a boy from my or my wife's background could not even imagine an act of that kind. I am convinced that vegetarianism, the backbone of which is *Ahimsa*, non-violence, is best for human society and that Hinduism greatly helps shape people to that way of life. The lessons learned during childhood days from one's elders go a long way toward shaping one as a vegetarian. Not only that, he is also one who hesitates to kill an animal for any cause.

I am a strict vegetarian and maintain excellent health at the age of 67. So, also is my wife, who is 60. I can say this about elderly relatives now in their 70s who have remained strict vegetarians. My mother again a strict vegetarian had lived in good health up to 92 years of age before breathing her last on January 7, 1993. Meat is not at all essential in one's diet for maintaining good health. My wife and I enjoy excellent health and remain very active mentally and physically. So, it is really vegetarianism that we must promote-left-right and centre....."

This clearly brings out the influence of social practices incorporated in oneself.

The Karma Angle

'*Karma*' is a Sanskrit word which means action or the act or doing something materially. Such material action brings back a reaction and binds us to the world. The law of *Karma* implies that every action of ours causes a reaction which is opposite in direction, that is directed towards us, bearing the same nature as our action. In simple words, if we cause pain and suffering to others, we must also endure pain and suffering. This law of *Karma* is deep-rooted in Hindu philosophy and now finds acceptance in the Western world as well.

How does the law of *Karma* apply in case of vegetarianism? If we kill animals for food we inflict cruelity and pain on those food-animals. In return, we shall have to endure pain and cruelty inflicted on us, if not in this world, then in the next world. A meat-eater however may question that he does not kill animals to eat but simply buys meat from the market. But his action or *Karma* leads to animals being killed. He in fact pays to the shopkeeper for killing of animals. If there is no buyer of meat, all meat shops will be closed down and killing of animals for food will be automatically stopped.

There is another argument that some people bring forward when killing of animals is criticized on grounds of cruelty. They argue that even plants have life in them, then why should we kill them for eating while sparing animals. This argument is refuted on various other grounds discussed in detail elsewhere in the book. First being, we have something to eat to live and while it is true that plants have life in them, they are not as sensitive and lively as animals are. The other argument is that God has given its verdict on the kind of food different species should eat by making their body suitable to particular kind of food. So, if a carnivorous animal, say lion, kills another animal for eating no question of ethics is involved. And when we compare the human anatomy we find that it compares more with herbivores than with carnivores. It implies that God has ordained man to eat plant food.

Thirdly, Hindu philosophy stresses upon austerity in the matter of food consumption. It says that we should eat only enough to survive and not eat more which in turn leads to bare minimum consumption of plants. This philosophy is very well summed up by Gandhiji in these words; *"Eat to live and not live to eat."*

Vedas say,

"Jivo jivasya jivanam"

i.e. 'one living entity is food for another in the struggle of existence'. So the problem is not to eliminate killing altogether but to avoid unwanted and unnecessary killings and to cause least suffering to other creatures.

Taking of life of any kind, even of plants is sinful according to Hindu religion but Krishna, the Supreme Controller, according to this religion offers a way-out. We offer food to Krishna and eating food after offering to the lord, we are freed from the sin. Eating such food is akin to a soldier killing during war time such food is called 'Prasada' and eating Prasada is not sinful. But we must offer vegetables, fruits and the kind to the Lord and not the meaty stuff. This is clearly mentioned in the *Bhagvad-Gita* wherein Krishna states, "offer me with love and devotion a fruit, a flower a, leaf or water and I will accept it."

Morality and Vegetarianism

To further the argument based on Hinduism, it may be said that any man who harbours feelings of *Ahimsa*, compassion, benevolence in his heart is quite unlikely to indulge in deeds that may cause pain to other living beings. It is so because human feelings determine human deeds. A morally just person following the Hindu ways of thinking is unlikely to take to eating of meat. According to studies, vegetarian population is less likely to indulge in anti-social behaviour.

Several Gurus and Swamis ot various sects that have appeared within the Hindu fold, like Radha Swamis, followers of Sai Baba, Asa Ram Bapu and the like have taken up the cause to take people away from meat-eating habits and lead them towards a vegetarian way of life. And their number is swelling all the time. They highlight the points that meat-eating undermines the equilibrium and the education of mind. It stimulates urges, cruelty and violence. A meat-eater's attitude is selfish and he finds enjoyment in giving pain to others. Here it will not be out of place to mention that a survey conducted on criminal in a prison revealed that 75 per cent of criminals were meat-eater and 25 per cent took vegetarian diet.

There have been records of people indulging in meat-eating and drinking before committing acts like rape and murder. Whether the correlation between the two is linear or else, is up to the judgment of the reader. The aim is not to be judgmental about anybody's eating practices but to present facts and let the readers decide for themselves.

Cow Worship

According to ancient scriptures, the original cow, Mother Surabhi, was one of the treasures churned from cosmic ocean, and the five products of the cow or the panch-gavya—milk, curd, ghee, urine and dung—were considered as purifying. The cow gets respect in the Hindu religion as mother because her milk is useful to human beings as that of natural mother.

The cow besides being worshiped has always played a big role in India's economy. Besides its milk, cow dung serves as an inexpensive fertilizer used in agriculture, by its underground processing, methane gas is produced which is used as a fuel for cooking. Cow dung is also a disinfectant and a cleansing agent. For all these reasons, Cow is a sacred animal for Hindus and is given protection against killing. This animal is called *aghnaya* which means "not to be killed."

It was probably to detain beef consumption in generations for moral as well as economic reasons (disguised as religion) that cow was given the status of mother and goddess in Hindu religion and culture.

The sages of ancient India had already recognized spirituality in animals and that was long before St. Francis was declared the pattern saint of animals. Vedic texts depict several incarnations of God in various animal forms. Popular among such are the boar, the tortoise, the fish and the horse. There are also incarnations in form of half man-half animal. However, the *Vedas* do not promote polytheism but hold firmly that these are the various forms of same one God.

Vedic scriptures also acknowledge the ability in animals to achieve exalted form of spirituality. In doing so, it is acknowledged that spirituality is not limited to human form or is not slave to any particular kind of external body but is associated with soul which keeps changing its abode from one body to another. This religious view-point views spirituality of all living beings in larger context of which vegetarianism is but a part.

All this leads us to believe that in any religion vegetarianism is the only way of living linked to eating and it links vegetarianism to morality and spirituality.

The Hindu Veda

As described earlier the history of Vegetarianism in India (and in Indian culture) goes down to our earliest ancestors. Indian Vedic-culture has been divided into early Vedic and later Vedic by the historians. But the original Vedic culture was quite different from contemporary Indian Culture or let's say, contemporary Hinduism; however, both old and new converge harmoniously in regard to vegetarianism. The *Vedas* have taught us of living in harmony with Nature and by killing any 'prani' (animal-rather say living being) we destroy this harmony, i.e., ecological balance as it is said in the *Vedas* that... "every part and parcel of nature is the creation of God and He is present in all forms of life."

Yajurveda (12:32) says, "You must not use your God-given body for killing God's creatures whether they are human, animal on whatever."

"Door of salvation is open for one who does not kill any living being, "(*Manusmriti*, 6:60) meaning that one should refrain from all sorts of violent acts (including eating of animals flesh) for such eating involves killing and leads to '*Karmic bandhan*' (bondage).

Maharaja Parikshit, last of the Vedic kings, is quoted to be saying that "only the animal killer cannot relish the message of the Absolute Truth."

The *Vedas* say that living soul transmigrates from body to body, from one species to the other until it reaches the human form, equipped with reason and sensibility and rationality. It is the human form of the soul which is able to know the 'Absolute Truth'. Charles Darwin is nearer to this concept of the Veda by propagating the theory of evolutionism.

So, being a rational animal, man should act rationally in every walk of life. The '*Vedas*' and the '*Gita*' describe the 'soul' as the source of consciousness and every living being possesses a soul. Lord Krishna, in the *Bhagvad-Gita*, says that it is the soul that activates the body of every living being. The '*Vedas*' principle of the 'Progressive evolutionism' says that a soul in a lower form than human, evolves automatically to the next higher species, ultimately arriving the highest form—human; and killing an animal interrupts its progressive evolution through the species. Similar is the explanation of Shrila Prabhupad, who, in his *Srimad Bhagvadgita* purports says, "All living beings have to fulfill certain duration for being encaged in a particular type of material body. They have to finish the duration allotted in a particular body before being promoted on evolved to another body. Killing an animal or some other living entity simply places an impediment in the way of completing his term of imprisonment in a certain body. One should, therefore, not kill any living body for one's sensual gratification for this will be taken as an interruption in this way to a living entity."

Man, being the animal of highest order, can attain spiritual perfection by his deeds and vision granted by Him. Lord Krishna explains in *Bhagvad-Gita* (5:18) that man's spiritual perfection beings when he starts seeing the same God in every soul or in all living beings. He says, "The humble sage, by virtue of true knowledge, sees with equal vision a learned and gentle brahmana, a cow, an elephant, a dog and an outcast."

The Vedic view point even acknowledges the ability of ordinary animals to achieve exalted states of spirituality. This is so because of the viewpoint that spirituality is not limited to the human form and that ultimately the external body is a temporary housing for the eternal soul, and the soul leaves this temporary have when she starts her journey towards progressive evolution. *Bhagvad-gita's* verses 27-28 of 13th chapter can be cited as examples that state as below,

> "He, who, sees that the Lord of all is ever the same in all that is immortal in the world of mortality, he sees the truth. And when a man sees that the God in himself is the same God in all, i.e. he hurts not himself by not hurting others. Then he goes indeed to the highest path."

The *Mahabharata* if full of the verses suggesting non-violence, non-injury and abstention from eating animal (flesh, some examples—"He, who desires to increase the flesh of his own body by eating flesh of other creatures, lives in misery in whatever species he may take his birth". (Anu : 115:47) "Who can be more cruel and selfish than he who augments his flesh by eating the flesh of innocent animals?" "Those who desire to possess good memory, beauty, long life with perfect health and physical, moral and spiritual strength, should strictly abstain from hurting, killing or eating animals."

Ahimsa, in all forms—*mansa, vachan* and *karmana* (through mind, speech and action)—is prohibited in the Hindu scriptures thus farming an essential part of Hindu culture as the *Mahabharata* teaches—"*Ahimsa* (non-violence) is the highest dharma (religion); *Ahimsa* is the best tapas; *Ahimsa* is the greatest gift, *Ahimsa* is the highest self-control, *Ahimsa* is the highest sacrifice, *Ahimsa* is the highest power; *Ahimsa* is the highest friend, *Ahimsa* is the highest truth, *Ahimsa* is the highest teachings," (*Mahabharata* 18:116:37-41) and because the same Almighty lives in every living soul, so "One should never to others do what one regards as injurious or hurting to one's own self. This is the rule of dharma." (*Mahabharata* 18:113:8).

Every Meal is a *Prasad*

It has been a traditional practice of Indian people to offer to God first whatever one has as meal, thank Him for His act of kindness of supplying him with food, and then start eating the ruminants of such offerings as *prasadam* (grace of God). This is a Vedic practice that before eating anything one should offer the food-stuff to God as sacrifice with full devotion and be grateful to Him for He is the nourisher of the world. This practice keeps us humble and reminds us of the noble thought *yatha ann tatha man* (whatever we eat,—pure or impure, good or bad, eatable or non-eatable-has is impact on our thought and action). In the *Bhagvad*-Gita (9.27) Lord Krishna says, "Offer unto Me all that you do, all that you give away, all that you eat as well as the austerities that you may perform should be done as an offering unto Me."

Thus, the Hindu religion, Hindu scriptures and culture all emphasize not only on vegetarianism but also spiritual equality of all living beings. And vegetarianism of Hinduism is not just a food-style but a lifestyle, a philosophy of life— not to hurt any one even by thoughts, by words or by actions, and much more.

Buddhism

Buddhism is other major religion of the Eastern world. In fact, it has the largest number of followers with China, the most populous nation following mainly this religion besides India also having a large number of Buddhists. Other nations having followers of Buddhism include Japan, Nepal, Sri Lanka, Bhutan, Myanmar, Hongkong, etc.

Buddhism originated in India and is an offshoot of Hinduism. Thus, it is natural for it to have influences of Hinduism on it. Buddhists also believe in the Law of *Karma* and hold that they will eventually suffer the consequences of their evil-doings.

Vegetarianism has always been central to Buddhism, which enshrines compassion to all living creatures. The Indian king Asoka (who reigned between 264-232 BC) converted to

Buddhism, shocked by the horrors of battle. Animal sacrifices were ended as his kingdom became vegetarian.

'Mercy' as Reason

Buddhist advocates of vegetarianism base their logic mainly on the reason of mercy. They hold that they cannot bear even the thought of eating flesh of living creatures. They also think on the lines that a vegetarian diet keeps the body and mind pure and to them purity is important in the way of self-cultivation.

Mercy is an essential feature of Buddhism and a person without mercy is incompatible with being a Buddhist. Being merciful makes a person better. A person having a merciful heart shows it up in all his doings and in all aspects of life but the simplest way to reflect it is by following the vegetarian diet.

If one spares a thought about the pain that an animal goes through while being slaughtered, skinned, dismembered and cooked, one is sure to be affected. Buddhism advocates such thoughts and Buddhists say that they are unable to bring themselves to eat the flesh of poor creatures by repeatedly imagining their plight. This is what they mean by mercy. Some popular non-vegetarian food varieties include cooking of animals like shrimp and crab. Meeting their end while being boiled in water is like being sent to hell, boiling. The desperate efforts they make to crawl or jump out, may move anybody who is watching the scene. But most of those who enjoy the bright red meat often do not witness the suffering the animals have to go through.

War is perhaps the worst kind of suffering that human race comes across. But wars are not fought every day. One war separates another by a margin of several years. But the war declared on animals goes on everyday. And to think these animals are reared so that they may go through the pain for pleasure of human beings is perhaps as inhuman an act as these can be.

Let me here recount the two stories on the theme of mercy that I read in a book sometime. First one goes like this:

Once a scholar named Chou Yu was cooking some eel to eat. He noticed that one eel was arching its body in such a way that while its head and tail remained inside the boiling soup, its body arched upward and above the level of soup. It remained thus till the eel died and fell inside. It was a strange occurrence. Chou Yu took that eel out and cut it open. To his surprise, he found a large number of eggs inside its belly. The reason now became obvious that eel was trying to protect its offspring. This brings out that animals like eel are also sensitive and have intelligence which makes their suffering all the more sinful for humanity.

Then there is another story. This story is given in Buddhist sutra.

A king of heaven got engaged in a war with a demon. None of the sides could beat the other. Finally the king of heaven led his solders back. On the way he saw the nest of a golden-winged bird on a tree. He thought, if the soldiers and chariots pass by here, the eggs in the nest will certainly fall to the ground and be scattered." So he ordered his soldiers back the same road by which they came. When demon saw them coming back, they were terrified and fled.

The sutra concludes the story thus, "If you use mercy to seek salvation, the lord of heaven will see it." The story reveals that mercy may seem of little value at a glance but its impact on fact is quite powerful. The Buddhist sutras make frequent mention of mercy as being a powerful instrument and a potent force. If a person with Buddhist learning wants to experience the power of mercy, he must be willing to indulge in mercy of the magnitude of turning the course of the thousands of chariots to save the eggs from falling on ground.

Large volumes have been written on Buddhist teachings regarding cause and compassion. In all those teachings the basic philosophy remains the same, "Good is rewarded with good and evil is rewarded with evil. Rewarding of good and evil is only a matter of time. We shall have pay back good or evil in the same coin, i.e., if we eat a piece of flesh we repay it by our piece of flesh; if we take a life, we have to lose a life for it at some stage. No action is done without a reaction to it."

The Surgama Sutra notes, "If we eat the flesh of living creatures, we are destroying the seeds of compassion. Contrary to it, if we do not eat the flesh of living creatures we are cultivating and irrigating the seeds of compassion."

Purifying Body and Mind

Buddhist argument on vegetarianism extends beyond mercy and causes and consequence concept and takes up the issue of body and mind becoming impure by consumption of meat. This concept gives the logic that all animals do not die in good health. Before death they secrete toxic substances. While eating flesh, we also take in disease-oriented micro-organism and toxins, etc. In comparison, vegetarian food is clean, fresh and healthy. Meat and meat products decay early whereas vegetables retain their nutritious values much longer. Another point is that decay in vegetables is clearly noticeable which not the case with meat.

There is a question facing vegetarianism. It is asked thus, "why can't you eat food items like onions and garlic?" On the issue Surangama Sutra says, "All living creatures seek here kinds of wisdom and should refrain from eating the 'five pungent'. These five pungent foods create lust if eaten cooked and if eaten raw they create rage." Further it says, "Even if someone can recite twelve sutras from memory, the god of heaven will disdain him if he eats pungent foods in this world because of his strong odour and uncleanliness, and will give distance themselves far from him." This means that pungent food arouse lust and cause temper to rise. In other words such foods corrupt the purity of body and mind. And if one's body and mind are not pure, Buddhism cannot help him purify them.

Another Buddhist sutra says, "That which has blood and flesh and blood will be rejected by gods and not eaten by saints, all in heaven distance themselves far from one who eats meat; his breath is foul—meat is not a good thing, meat is not pure, it is born in evil and spoils in merit and virtues, it is rejected by all the gods and saints."

In a way initiation into Buddhism begins at the dining table. One must first purify his body and mind by adopting vegetarianism and then and only then should one attempt to become a Buddhist.

Dr. Walsh, an Englishman, promoter of vegetarianism, says, "To prevent human bloodshed one must start at the dinner table."

Buddhism appreciates every life and killing of animals is against Buddha Dharma. Vegetarianism is the basic foundation of Buddhism. Buddhist philosophy does all to promote vegetarianism though all Buddhists are not vegetarians. This is the reality of their world as of all other. After all we cannot have a utopian world but a practical world. But all efforts must be made to change the world for better. Buddhists believe that Buddha Maitreya is the next Buddha and Maitreya will come several billion years later. But in view of prevailing condition, he is needed here before that time to spread the teachings of vegetarianism. It is a continuous struggle of Buddhism to make people convert to vegetarianism.

Nirvana

Vegetarianism in Buddhism is based on the Buddhist doctrine of '*Nirwana*' or '*Moksha*' i.e. salvation which is based on the Hindu philosophy of the equality of living beings and the belief that the same 'Soul' is present in all living entities. As in Hinduism, it is believed also in Buddhism that a person can get rid of the cycle of death and rebirth by means of his good *'karma'* (works or actions); he can achieve enlightenment through good thought and meditation. Mahatma Buddha had set-out to ease the *'dukkha'* (the sorrows) of living beings; he had started his journey to save others from agony. Buddha, when a child, had saved an injured goose from a poacher, it was out of compassion and mercy he had for any and every living being. So Buddhism in based on the principles of compassion, mercy and salvation and a Buddhist should act on this line of thought and action.

In order to achieve *'Nirvana'* or salvation one should save his own soul from sin and its consequences; and a true Buddhist is he who saves others from 'dukha'. So, an action of saving others from *'dukkha'* is a virtue, not afflicting others in any way is a virtue and a virtuous soul is always rewarded with 'salvation.'

'Save yourself so that you can save others' is the true spirit of an *Arahat*; *Arahat* is a true Buddhist who obeys *'panchsheela'*—the five principles—of Buddhism, and the first 'sheela' of Buddhism is vegetarianism. Without being a vegetarian, how can one save oneself from afflicting others; how can one save other from *'dukkha'*? By way of adopting vegetarianism we do save ourselves from *'dukkha'* and we also save other living beings from *'dukkha'* Certainly vegetarianism is the basic principle of Buddhism, *Bodhisatva* and *Arahat* since the first 'sheela' of true Buddhism in *"Ahimsa"*—"Do no kill." And eating meat without killing or afflicting other animal is simply impossible. So, a humble suggestion for every person who wants to enjoy the Buddhist way of life and enter into the realm of knowledge and mercy of the Buddha, he must begin at the dinning table. The pain of creatures on way to out dinning table is not some fanciful concoction, it is excruciatingly real. Our food creatures like live shrimp and crab, which are popular these days, suffer through the greatest pain one can imagine. They cross through a boiling hell when cooked in water or fried in oil. Their desperate but doomed efforts to crawl or jump out betray the unbearable sufferings they experience. Finally they give their life in extreme sorrow as they turn bright red. An unimaginable painful end. How can one have the heart to eat the flesh of poor creatures who have suffered the pain of being slaughtered, skinned, dismembered and cooked? Bringing ourselves to not eating the flesh of these poor creatures is an expression of mercy, mercy being the most essential element of Buddhism. Preventing the suffering of living beings by not using their flesh to satisfy our taste buds and hunger is the minimal expression of mercy and compassion we can offer.

Jainism

Jainism is one of the oldest religions practiced in India. Archeological findings suggest that the religion flourished 5000 to 8000 years ago amongst the people of Indus valley civilization. Today Jains form a small religious community in India. They follow a strong moral code of conduct in their lifestyles and strictly adhere to vegetarianism. People of Jain community are generally economically strong, healthy and respected people in the society. They are perhaps the best example of success of vegetarianism. They show no signs of dietary deficiencies which are often wrongly associated with vegetarian diet.

Code of Conduct

As already mentioned, Jains follow a rather tough and disciplined code of conduct in their living. Non violence of thought as well as of action is the fundamental basis of Jainism. The religion preaches truthfulness, equal rights for all irrespective of caste, race, gender, age and religion, compassion for all living beings, vegetarianism, not to steal, etc. These all teachings are different manifestations of the principle of non-violence. The Jains follow the 24 *Tirthankaras* in tradition. Tirthankaras are the master preachers who appeared at different periods of time and enlightened the path of salvation. The most recent of their *Tirthankaras* was Lord Mahavira who lived and preached during the period 599-527 B.C. Jainism is traced back to Mohenjo-Daro and Harappa civilization about 8000 years back. This reveals that/ vegetarianism is that practice of much old if not more.

Jainism and Vegetarianism

Though not vegans, Jains are strict vegetarians, and vegetarianism in Jainism dates back to the Indus valley (Mohenjo-Daro, Harappa and Lothal) civilization 5000 to 8000 years ago, when this religion flourished. Jains follow strict diet codes that restrict even the use of many products of plant origin within the vegetarian regime.

Jainism is a scientific way of life which recognises plants as a form of life and gives a scientific definition of Vegetarianism, its limitations and necessity for the survival of the human race. Without any apparent dietary deficiencies, Jains are a living example of the success of a vegetarian diet farming a community of healthy, accomplished and mostly upper middle-class of the India of the Indian society.

Vegetarianism of Jainism in based on absolute non-violence of thought and action which happens to be the very basic principle of Jainism. Including vegetarianism, truthfulness, equal right for all-irrespective of cast and creed, gender and age, race and religion-compassion and love for all living beings etc. are but different manifestation of the principle of non-violence.

Realizing that human beings must eat to survive and derive nutrition Jainism permits foods procured from plants only for human consumption. Still there are strict dietary codes of practice recommended for day to day living on the consumption of plant-based diet. These include prohibition on the consumption of some vegetables and fruits, restrictions on the way of procurement of produce (e.g. potatoes not be procured and eaten in the rainy season as they grow underground and harbour numerous tiny creatures), restrictions on times and livings etc.

Consumption of fig family fruits is not permitted as these fruits are inhabited by species of wasps specific to each; i.e. the entire life cycle of the wasps is completed within the fig and its sister fruits. It is a fact established by modern day science that some kind of wasps compete their life cycle within the fig and her sister fruits and these fig family fruits contain in them the remnants of the eggs and the dead wasps.

The Jain concept of vegetarianism has unconditional compassion and reverence for all forms of life. A comparative study of religions presented at the World Environment Congress in U.K. pronounced Jainism the most eco-friendly religion of the world. It was stated that if the whole world could think and live the Jain's way, there would be no environmental problems and extinction of species. Jainism put vegetarianism not just to dinning table, but makes it a holistic lifestyle.

Jainism provides a scientific basis to the definition of vegetarianism. Jains recognize plants as life form and detail our the necessity of vegetarianism for the betterment of humanity as well as its limitations. Like other religions and cultures that promote vegetarianism, Jainism also practices vegetarianism for reasons of compassion and non-violence.

However, concept of non-violence has much deeper meaning for Jains than others. Jains long back acknowledge that plants have life. Now the question arises that if plants have life it is not violent to eat plant-based foods. Jain argues to this question is quite logical and clearly.

Jains consider five physical senses as attributes of life, namely, touch, taste, smell, sight and hearing. All life forms are classified by them on this basis. Higher the life form, more the senses. Lower the life form, lesser the senses. Examples are given to this kind of classification. The highest life form existing on the earth is the human beings. Humans have all the five physical senses. Lower forms include mosquitoes with four senses—touch, taste, smell and sight; lice with three sense: touch, taste and smell earth worm with two senses-touch and taste. Plants form the lower life form and they are sensitive to touch only. Now it is an established fact their man needs nutrition for survival for Jains, this nutrition must come from the lowest life form, hence they approve of plant-based food only. In arriving at this conclusion, Jains of ancient times have made a great contribution to the modern life sciences providing basis for study of evolution of living beings.

Even while approving consumption of plant-based foods, several restrictions are placed in order to preserve plant life. Such restrictions include prohibition on consumption of certain fruits and vegetables, restriction on procurement of produce, observing timings, fasting, being selective in choosing occupations, etc. These prohibitions are discussed below.

Restrictions on Food Selection

Jains are quite fussy when it comes to food selection and all this has to do with non-violence, hygiene or conservation of environment. They in fact, have practices and taught to others centuries ago the things we are learning through modern sciences only now.

Vegetables and fruits that grow underground are not consumed by orthodox Jains. The logic here is that to procure such produced the whole plant is destroyed as we pull it out of the ground. Besides, other microorganisms living around the plants roots are also destroyed. Fruits and vegetables from plants should be plucked only when they are ready to fall from the plant. Better still, fallen fruits are preferred for consumption. Grains are recommended for procurement only when their pods are dry and dead. Cutting of green trees for procurement is prohibited. Procurement should be done to the bare minimum level without any waste. This ways Jains set an example in the conservation of plants life.

This apart Jainism follows the practice of fasting twice every fortnight, on the eighth and fourteenth day of the full and new moon cycles of the lunar calendar. During fasting only foods prepared from grains is consumed and green vegetables and fruits are avoided.

Jains today have somewhat relaxed the restrictions on root vegetables and fruits and started consuming them for social convenience. This does not take them away from vegetarianism and they remain strict on vegetarian diet as they earlier were.

Multi-seeded fruits and vegetables like brinjal, guava etc. are not consumed by conventional Jains. It is so because they sometimes contain worms in them. If some Jains do eat such vegetables, they are cut and thoroughly cleaned first. Common practice of cooking the brinjal by roasting the whole brinjal is not followed by Jains. They also avoid eating cauliflower and broccoli as they have velvety surfaces and sometime organisms are likely to get stuck in them.

Jackfruit is another example of specific restriction. It is avoided as it bleeds on cutting and looks like meat after cooking. Mushrooms and fungus are avoided as they grow in unhygienic conditions. Cabbage and green leafy vegetables are thoroughly cleaned leaf by leaf and then cooked as there is possibility of living organisms residing in between the leaves.

Timing of Consumption

Another major restriction concerns **timing** of cooking and eating. Food must be cooked and consumed between dawn and dusk. Jains do not consume even water before dawn and after dusk. This practice is carried from ancient times where there was no adequate means of lighting. In dark, animals might be killed by fire. Such animals could be hiding in wood or coal or could be in the food articles to be cooked. This practice is followed even today by Jains. While eating food small insects are likely to fall in the food being eaten and consumed by mistake. Also going to bed after consuming food is not a healthy practice. And Jains follow the practice of sleeping early as also getting up early. (Practically speaking this practice of eating before sunset helps in proper digestion of food before person falls asleep and thus keeps the system in perfect order)

Jains do not consume food cooked in shops and restaurants but consume food cooked at home only. Stale food is not taken and fresh food is cooked every day. This is done to avoid wastage and also for reasons that insects may creep into the food kept overnight. Growth of bacteria in the cooked food kept overnight is also a reason for this. Fresh food is always good from the viewpoint of health too.

As regards water, it is advised that water be filtered through three layers of home-spun cotton cloth. On becoming wet, cotton cloth behaves as a cotton pad; water passes through it by the process of surface tension; and not through gaps between fiber if synthetic fiber is used. This ensures effective filtration and elimination of suspended particles and microorganisms present in water. This method does not ensure the removal of dissolved impurities. But then, in ancient times such impurities were not in vogue and are a recent phenomenon. Even today all the doctors, health conscious beings are taking and preferring filter water only. Otherwise, the method is quite convenient and cheap method of cleaning water and is used even today. The cloth used for filtration should be rinsed in a river or well to return the microorganisms to their natural habitat. This is a great example of coexistence of human being with their environment and caring even for microbes.

Jains allow use of milked dairy products provided that they are procured and made according to the laid-down rules. Before milking a cow, its calf must be allowed to suckle about one-third of the expected yield. The milk should be boiled within 48 minutes of milking and consumed within 24 hours. Yoghurt consumption is allowed only if prepared daily from freshly boiled milk using the leaf of a particular plant and consumed within 24 hours. Yoghurt prepared by using previous day's Yoghurt is considered stale and is not considered edible. Cheese also is considered stale and not eaten.

Christianity

Opinions differ on the stand of Christianity on the issue of vegetarianism. Consumption of non-vegetarian diet is widely prevalent in Christian society and there seem to be no religious restriction in place on consumption of such diet. However, when we dig deeper into Christian ideology we find that though contradicting stands appear on different occasions, yet non-violence, compassion and love for animals is strongly advocated. Let us look at these aspects and how they were advocated in earlier period of Chirstianity.

Early Christianity and Vegetarianism

If we look back early period of Christianity, we find a large number of vegetarians among them both in the leadership class as well as in ordinary citizenry. Augustine, though not a vegetarian himself hold those in high esteem who abstain from meat and wine. Here it may be noted that in general Christians need not necessarily be vegetarians.

Of those leaders of the early Church who were vegetarians, the name of James, the brother of Jesus, may be mentioned. He was evidently raised as a vegetarian

(Ecclesiastical History 2.23). Why would Jesus' parents have raised James as a vegetarian unless they themselves were also vegetarian and also raised Jesus as a vegetarian? Other famous vegetarian Christians included Basil the Great, John Chrycostom Arnobius, Tertullia and Jerome. *Euse Das* states that all the apostles abstained from meat and wine (proof of Gospel 3.5). A question that we come across here is that was Jesus a vegetarian. On the evidence of James, brother of Jesus, having been brought up as a vegetarian we may presume that Jesus was brought up as a vegetarian too as same parents would on support their two children on different diets basing exceptional reasons. But on Biblical evidence this question is not easy to answer. Evidently James fed bread and fish to the multitude causing us to believe that he approved of eating fish. But his compassion towards animal (Mathew 12: 10-12) hints at his being a vegetarian. New Testament takes contradictory stand on the issue seeming to support vegetarianism at one point and oppose it at another.

It appears from Paul's letter that church in early Christianity did not take any rigid stand on the eating of food. While many Christians practiced vegetarianism, the church did not insist on its practice. "As for the one who is weak in faith, welcome him, but not for disputes over opinions. One believed he may eat anything, the weak man eats only vegetables" says Paul (Romans 14: 1-2). Paul advocates patience between the meat-eaters and the vegetarians. "Eat whatever is sold in the meat market without raising any question on grounds of consciences." Says Paul (Icorinthians 10: 25)

Some early Christians notably the Jewish Christians opposed Paul's stand. They were vegetarians and believed that all Christians should practice vegetarianism.

Jewish Christians on Vegetarianism

In the opinion of Jewish Christians, Jewish didn't come to start a new religion but spread the message of simple living and non-violence. To them, Jesus didn't overturn the Jewish law but preached the correct practice of Jewish Law as He understood it; a law of advocating simple living and non-violence. Jesus was a prophet in the eyes of Jewish Christians and loyal to the law. But he interpreted law to reach radical conclusions. The Jewish Christians therefore took to simple living, pacifism and vegetarianism.

'Ebonites' were the chief Jewish Christians group. The Jewish Christian writings like—*The Clementine Homilies, the Recognitions of Clement* and the *Panarion of Epiphanins,* give us knowledge about their beliefs. 'Ebonite' is the terms derived from a Hebrew word which means 'the poor'. 'Ebonites' called themselves, 'the poor' and traced their poverty back to the primitive Christian community which shares all their possessions in common. Thus, there was no concept of private property and community owned everything. And communities cared for every one. As already mentioned Jewish Christians are vegetarians and lived in non-violence. They were pacifists and were opposed to wars and killing. This fact finds mention several times in *The Recognitions* (1.70-71, 2: 36, 3. 42)

Frequent mention is found of the Jewish Christians' opposition to meat-eating and sacrifice of animals in the temples in both the *Homilies* and *Recognition.* The Homilies state their strong opposition to killing of animals (3.45) and their condemnation of meat-eaters (7.4, 7.8). Support of vegetarianism and opposition to animal sacrifice is a distinctive feature of the Jewish community which is brought out in various Christian documents.

Regarding animal sacrifice it may be mentioned that in ancient times the temple in Jerusalem was quite different from a modern church. It resembled more to Jerusalem shop than a worship place. People brought animals there to sacrifice and priests kept most of the meat. This way the priests were benefited economically. This priestly sanction to the ghastly practice which had no religious sanction angered the Jewish Christian. Jesus says, "I require mercy not sacrifice" (Mathew) 9.13, 12.7). Ebontite gospels also quotes Jesus thus, 'I have come to abolish the sacrifices and if you cease not from sacrificing, my wrath will not cease from you." (Pamarion 30.16.5). Jesus called the temple a 'den of robbers'. He emphasized that God did not need sacrificing. During His last days, Jesus went to the temple and disrupted the animal sacrifice business.

The end result was that Jesus was crucified by the Romas possibly, it was the disruption of animal sacrifice business and its interpretation as a threat to public order that was the most important reason of death of Jesus.

The cause (of disruption of animal sacrifice business) was definitely essential for Jesus's message and that is only possible reason for Jesus to risk his life.

Vegetarianism as a practice got abandoned because of popularity of Paul's letters among the early Christians. The early leadership like Peter and John was opposed to Paul but teachings of Paul kept on gaining popularity. Paul's stand on vegetarianism (it is optional for individuals and in no way a restriction in Christianity) led the Church and Christians on the path of meat-eating.

New Testament with editors distorting it to their own view points, distorted the stand of Jesus on animals. This led to the loss of religion that Jesus preached and modern Christianity diverted from it.

However, winds of change are being sensed in the Western world, the real world of Christianity and several of them are seen returning to vegetarianism as has been discussed elsewhere in this book.

Islam

The religion of Islam has always regarded animals as a special part of God's creation. *The Qur'an,* the Hadith and the history of Islamic civilization offer many examples of kindness, mercy and compassion for animals. The following quotes from none other than the Prophet Mohammad make this amply clear.

The Prophet Mohammad (peace be upon him) as narrated by Abdallah bin Amru, in Bukhari and Muslim collections:

"Whosoever is kind to the creatures of God, is kind to himself."

The Holy Prophet (peace be upon him) said on the subject of caging of birds:

"It is great sin for man to imprison those animals which are in his power."

(Muslim)

The Holy Prophet (peace be upon him) forbade the beating and branding of animals. Once he saw a donkey branded on its face and said:

"May Allah condemn the one who branded it".

(Muslim)

The Holy Prophet Muhammad (peace be upon him) was asked by his companions if kindness to animals was rewarded in life here-after. He replied,

"Yes, there is a meritorious reward for kindness to every living creature."

(Bukhari)

There are numerous Islamic laws forbidding performing of vivisection on a live animal. (Al-Muthia). Ibn Umar reported the Holy Prophet (peace be upon him) as having condemned those who mutilate any part of an animal body while it is alive (Ahmad and other authorities).

In the eyes of Islam, all creatures on the earth are sentient beings,

"There is not an animal, nor a bird that flies on its wrings but they are communities like you."

(The Quran, 6: 38)

On food, Islamic views are thus reflected,

> "Food should be prepared from only lawful ingredients. Pork, alcohol, anything containing gelatine taken from a pig, sweep made with alcohol, blood, animals such as snake and frog...... unlawful to consume"

(Morals and Manners in Islam—A Guide to Islamic Adaab)

Though there is no direct reference to Vegetarianism, the kindness that Islam shows towards animals should be taken as a broad enough hint as a tilt of Islam, the religion towards vegetarianism. However like Christians, majority of Muslims are inclined towards non-vegetarian diet. But if the Islamic viewpoint is highlighted in the right perspectives chances are that more Muslims might switch to vegetarianism.

Some more sayings of Prophet Mohammad (Peace be upon him)

"Fear God, in treating dumb animals and ride them when they are fit to be ridden and get off them when they are tired."

"An adulteress passed by a dog at a well; and the dog was holding out his tongue from thirst, which was near killing him, and the woman drew off her boot and tied it to the end of her garment, and drew water for the dog and she was forgiven for that act."

"A woman was punished for a cat, which she tied till it died from hunger. She gave the eat nothing to eat, nor did she set it at liberty, so that it might find some food."

Are there rewards for our doing good to quadrupeds and giving them water to drink?" Muhammad said, "Verily there are heavenly rewards for any act of kindness to a animal."

"Verily God hath one hundred loving kindnessess one of which He hath sent down amongst man, quadrupeds and every moving thing upon the face of the earth; by if they are kind to each other and forgive one another; and by it the animals of the wilds are kind to their young! and God hath reserved ninety nine loving kindness by which He will be graciou to His creatures on the last day."

A man came before the Rasul with a carpet and said, "O Rasul! I passed through a wood and heard the voices of the young of birds; and I took and put them into my carpet; and their mother came fluttering round my head, and I uncovered the young, and the mother fell down upon them, then I wrapped them up in carpet; and there are the young which I have." Then the Rasul said, "put them down". And when he did so, their mother joined them; and Muhammad said, "Do you wonder at the affection of the mother towards her young? I swear by him who hath sent me, verily God is more loving to his creatures than the mother to these young birds. Return them to the place from which ye took them, and let their mother be with them."

The lower animals were not excluded from the benefits of the Prophet's all embracing love. It is recorded of him that when being on journey, he alighted at any place; he did not say his prayers until he had unsaddled his camel, a piece of animal conduct which puts us strongly in mind of the famous last lines of Coleridge's.

Ancient Mariner;

"He prayeth well, who loveth well.

Both man and bird and beast.

He prayeth best, who loveth best.

All things both great and small,

For the dear God who loveth us,

He made and loveth all."

There is nothing surprising in this loving kindness of the Prophet, for as he himself put it:

'Whoever is kind to his creatures, Allah is kind to him.

"All His creatures are Allah's family, for their subsistence is from Him; therefore the most beloved unto Allah is the person who does good to Allah's family;

'Who is the most favoured of Allah? He from whom the greatest good cometh to his creatures.'

"Do you love your creator? Then love your fellow creatures first."

The Prophet often insisted upon the rights of animals. He said,

"Fear God in respect of these dumb animals; ride them when they are fit to be ridden and get off when they are tired."

Indeed, as a Musalman writer assures us in the *Quran* animal life stands on the same footing as human life in the sight of God:

There is no beast on earth nor bird which flirth with its wings but the same is a people like unto you (mankind)—unto the Lord shall they return." (*Quran* VI, 38).

In one of his *jehads* the prophet found that a woman had been killed; thereupon he prohibited the killing of women and children.

As pointed out by D.S. Margoliouth, 'the Prophet forbade the employment of, living birds as targets for marksman and remonstrated with those who ill-treated their camels. When some of his followers had set fire to an anthill he compelled them to extinguish it. No more was the evil eye to be propitiated by the blinding of a certain proportion of the heard. No more was the rain to be conjured by tying burning torches to the tails of oxen and letting them loose among the cattle. Horses were not to be hit on the cheek and their manes and tails were not be cut, the former being meant by nature for their warmth, and the latter as a protection against flies. Asses were not to be branded or hit on the face. Even the cursing of cocks and camels was discouraged. When a common vowed to sacrifice her camel if it brought her safely to her destination, the Prophet ridiculed this mode of rewarding the beast's services and released her from her vow.'

The Prophet was never tired of dwelling upon the beauty of meekness. He said:

'God is mild and is fond of mildness and he giveth to the mild what he withholds from the harsh;

'Whoever is without mildness is without goodness.'

Meekness and modesty are two branches of Iman.

There is no accomplishment like an aimable disposition.

Religion of Peace

Islam is basically and historically a religion of Peace-Non-Violence, *Ahimsa, Adam-Tashaddud.* The very ward 'Islam'

(Arabic root 'Salm') means 'peace', 'making of peace' 'submission' 'resignation'-*'atmsahamarpan'* : Peace with the Maker and the whole creation.

Peace with Man, as contemplated in Al-Karan is the means of attaining Peace with God, the end. Peace with God is attained through good deeds done to our fellow beings including the subhuman. So, in *Sura Al-Baqara,* we have:

"Balaman' aslama wajhahu lillahi wa huwa muhsinum falahu ajruhu inda Rabbihi wala Knaufun alaihim wala hum yahzanun: Yea, whosever resigns himself to the will of Allah, and he is the doe of good to others, there will be reward for him from his Lord and he shall not grieve."-2:112.

So, the well-known Hadith (Traditions: sayings of the Prophet Muhammed) is: *"Khairun nasi main yan fa'unannas* : The best of man is he who does the greatest good to humanity."

In verse 2:62 we read: *"Innaal Iadhina amanu walledhina hadu wan-nasare was sabi'ina man amana billahi wal-yawmiakhiri wa amila salihan falahum ajuhum inda Robbihiml* verily those who believe (in Allah) and those who are Jews and the Christians and the Sabians—whoever believe in Allah and the Last Day (Retribution) and do good acts, they shall have their reward from their Lord (Rab)."

In *Sura An-Nisa*:

Wa-man ahsanu dinam mim-man aslama wajahu lillahi was hua muhsinun: And who can be better in religion than one who submits his own self to Allah and does good to others." (4:125)

Such a man, irrespective of his faith, is in the Karanic sense a 'Muslim'-'a maker of peace, Peace-Non-Violence is the massage and the central teaching of Islam.

So, the great German philosopher poet (Goethe) reading the *Koran* exclaimed: "If this is Islam, then every thinking man among us is, in fact, a Muslim."

In the Hadith of the Holy Prophet we have "Muslim is one from whose hands, tongue and limbs everyone is Safe":

"Verily, he is not a Muslim, who fills up his stomach, while his neighbours are starving": "The smallest service, for even a minute, is for more valuable than spending the whole of a year in prayers."

Islam is "a life to be lived in present." So, in *Sura Al-Baqara*, verse 2:177, we have the definition of Muslim, the Righteous":

Laisal Birra an tuwallu ujuhakum qilealal mashriq wal maghribi wa lakinnal birra man amana billahi wa yawmil akhiri wal malaikatiwal kitabi wan nabiyina wa atal mala ala hubbihi Zawil qurba wal yatama wal masakina wabnas—sabili was sailina wa fir riqabi wa aqamas salata wa ataz—zakata wal mufoona biahdihim iza ahudu was—subirina fil ba sayi waddarayi wa hinal basi wodaikal iadhina sadaqu woolaika humid muttaqoon:

It is not righteousness that you turn your faces (in prayer) towards the east or the west; but righteousness is of him who believes in God; and in the Hereafter (Akhirat) and in the Help and Guidance from Allah (angel); and in all the Scriptures; and in the Prophets: who giveth money for God's sake unto his kindred and unto orphans and the poor and the strangers and those needy who ask; and for the (redemption) of captives: who is constant at prayers and gives alms; and of those who perform their covenant when they have covenanted; and who behave themselves patiently in hardship and adversity and in times of distress: These are they that are the righteous (*muttaqi*) and the true (Muslim)."

In Sura Al-Hujurat, verse 49:13, we read: "*Inna akamakum indallahi atqukum* : Verily the most honoured of you in the sight of Allah is he who is the most righteous of you."

"Blind in this life, blind in the Hereafter" so says Al-Karan: *"We man Kana fi hajihi a,ma wahna fil akhirati a,ma."* (17: 72, Sura *Bani-Israil.*)

In Al-*Koran* the God of Islam is named *As'-salam*-the cause of Peace. Paradise (*Jannat*) is described as *Darus-salam* the Abode of Peace, *Shantiniklтan:* and defined as *salaman – salama* Peace, Peace (Sura Waqia, 56:25). In *Sura Yaseen* we have:

Inna ashabul-jannatil yawma fi shughulim fakihoon: Verily the companions of the Garden (*Jannat*) shall that Day have joy in all that they do 36:55."

The final Goal, 'Bliss of the Hereafter' (*Jannat*) is summed up and described as the very word PEACE, 'Word of Go'; in *Sura Yaseen,* verse 36:58; "*Salamun: quawlan mir Rabbir Raheen: (Jannat)* is Peace! Verily the word from the Most Merciful Lord." So, in the Holy Bible, St. John, 1:1, we read: "In the beginning was the word, and the Word was with God, and the word *was* God."

In Sura Furqan, verse 25:63, we read: "*Waibadur Rahmanillazina yamahuna alal ardi hownow wa iza khatabahumul jahillona qalu salamo:* The servants of the Merciful (Allah) are they that walk upon the earth softy: and when the ignorant speak unto them, they reply (greeting) 'Peace'.

Verse 25:75-76 say: "*Wulaika yujzawnal ghaurfata bima sabaru wa yulaqquna feeha tahiyyatawn wa salama khalidina feea hasumal, mustaqarawn wa muqama:* They (the righteous) shall be rewarded for their perseverance (sabr); and they shall be accosted in Paradise with welcome and salutation of Peace: For herein ever a fair abode and (peaceful resting place."

In the Traditions of the Holy Prophet Muhammad (*Hadith*) we have: "Faith in God is a wall against Violence." Non-Violence was the basis of the Holy Prophet Muhammad's mission. He constantly adhered to the injunction of the Karan of calling people gently towards the new Faith, Islam. The famous sermon, delivered in the hour of victory by the Prophet to the assembled people, after the full of Mecca, begins by a declaration of the natural Equality and Brotherhood of Man, and then proceeds. "Descendants of Koraish how do you think I shall act towards you?" "With kindness and pity' gracious brother and nephew" was the reply. The Holy Prophet assured: "I shall speak to you as Joseph spoke unto his brothers. I shall not reproach you today: God will forgive. He is Most Merciful and compassionate".

What a Superb Example of Non-violence

In *Sura Yaseen*, 36: 63-64, we have the opposite-*Jahannam*:

"Hajihi *Jahannam*ul lati Kuntum tu-adoon. Islawhal Yawma : This is the Hell of which you were repeatedly warned: Embrace ye the Fire this Day."

Peace with the Maker and Man (including the sub-human) is the Keystone of Islam, the Universal Religion of Love.

In *Sura Al-Baqara*:

"Kulu amanna biilahi wanaa unjila ilaina wama unjila ila Ibrahima wa Ismaila wa Ishaga wa Yakuba wal asbati wama wooti ya Musa was Isa wa ma wooti yan nabiyuna mir Rabbihim la nufarriqu baina ahadim mintum wa nahnu lahu muslimoon :

In 37:181 we have : "Wa Salamun allal mursaleen : And peace be to all the Prophets." In earlier verses of the same sura we have expressions of Peace and salutations'; to Abraham, Moses and other Prophets singly, and, through them, to all mankind.

So, in 21:92 we read : *'Inna hadhiti ummatukum* ummataw *wahidah* : Verily this Brotherhood of yours is a single Brotherhood." Again, in 2:213 (repeated in other verses) we have: "kanan-nasu *ummatwan wahidah* : Mankind was but one single nation-brotherhood."

All Prophets of God are referred to in Al-*Koran* as 'Muslim', and the religion preached by them as 'Islam': *Innad-dina indallahil islam* : The religion before Allah is Islam,-submisindallahil islam : The religion before Allah is Islam,-submission to His will-(3 :19). Al-*Koran* says: "Abrahm was not a Jew nor Christian, but he was an upright man, a Muslim; and he was not one of the polytheists: *Ma Kana Ibrahimu yahu-diyawn wala narraniyawn wa lakin kana hanifam musliman wama-kana minal-mushrikin"-3:67.*

My Islam would therefore, include the religion the Bhagavat *Gita*, and of the Lord Jesus Christ, and of Abraham and Moses, and in fact of all the Prophets.

Islam is natural religion of man. In Sura Ar-Rum (30:30): *"Fitratal-lahil-lati fataran naste alai-ha* : Allah created man in the natural religion." This verse, according to the celebrated Abu Huraira, companion of the Holy Prophet Muhammed was recited by the Prophet while delivering his famous Hadith (Tradition): "Every child is born, pure and sinless, in the natural religion of Islam; but afterwards it is his parents who make him a Jew or a Christian or a Magian-(Al. Hazrat Iman Bokhari).

When a Muslim meets any person he greets him with *Assalamu alaikum* : May peace be unto you. In Al-*Koran*, 4:86;

"Wa iz hui yitum bitahiyatin fahaiyu bi – ahsana minha awrudduha: And when others greet you, return the greeting with a better greeting." It is enjoined in Al-*Koran* that, if an enemy of opponent greets a Muslim, he (Muslim) should greet him in return. Verse 8:61 *"Wa in janahu lis-salmi fajnah loha wa tawakkal alallahi*: But if the enemy incline towards peace do thou also incline towards peace, and trust in Allah." In 4: 94,*"Wala taqulu liman alqa ilaikumus Salana lasta mu'mina* : And say not to any one who offers you salutation : thou art none of a Believer ?" Again, in 25: 63:

"And those are the servants (*abid*) of Allah, who walk on the earth with modesty: and even if a fool addresses him, he greets him, in return, saying 'peace not thee"! *(lalu Salama*). The Holy Prophet always followed this golden rule and was well-known for ideal and unique modesty and meekness. Islam is essentially a religion of peace, Non-violence. "Blessed are the meek : for they shall inherit the earth"-St. Mathew 5:5

In Sura Hujarat 49:13, we read :

"Ya ayyuhan nasu inna khalaqnakum min dhakarium wa untha wa-ja alnakum shu'kbawn wa qabaila litaarafu inna akramakum indallahi atqakum innallaha alimun Khabir : O'ye Man! We created you from a single pair of a male and a female, and made you into nations and tribes, *that ye may know each other-not that ye may despise each other.* Verily the most honoured of you in the sight of Allah is who is the most righteous of you : And Allah is well acquainted with all things."

In reality, there are only two distinc and diverse basic classes among mankind, the male and the female, (as we read also in verse 49 : 13 of *Al-Hujarat*), and out of the ir union in love, Man is born and sustained; and families, tribes and nations spring up and grow an units of society. Unity of Man is born out of the apparent diversity. That is the purpose of God – the Law of God.

Sura *Yunus*, verse 10 : 99, says :

"Wa-lau Sha'a rabbuka la'amana man fil-ardi Kulluhum jamia. Afanta tukrihun-nasa hatta yakunu mu'mineen :

If it had been the Lord's Will, they would all have believed in God,-all who are on the earth. Wilt thou than compel mankind against their will to believe?"

Let me quote from the Cultural Problem (Oxford Pamphlet).

"In my opinion, to seek unity in diversity and to accept that there will ever be differences in religious thinking, is our best aim. In Al-*Koran* we have the truth that, if Allah had willed, He could have so made Man as to have one single religion; but His will is to put mankind to test as to how man will use his own intelligence and discretion (free will). It seems, the diversity of human thought is embodied in the conception of God's creation itself; and in other matters too, such diversity is in consonance with natural sequence."

Let us accept that all religions have a right to live. Standing on the broad vantage-ground of Brotherhood, let us study all religious principles and respect them that in times of yore, the Sufis and saints of India had, by love and sympathy, conquered others, is manifest that they followed the above principle; and in the future, India will solve, through such noble thanking, her cultural problem."

(Re-translated from Bengali version in Dr. Suniti Kumar Chatterji's Bharat Sanskriti, 1944-Sir Abdul Qadir).

Love of man, as preached in Al-*Koran*, includes love of the sub-human. In Sura Aman '(cattle), we read in verse 6:38 :

"Wa-ma-min dabbatin fil-ardi wa-lajta'yirin yatiru bi-jana haihi illa umamum amthalukum Ma farratna fil-kitabi min shaiyin thumma ila Rab-bihim yuhsharoon :

There is not an animal that lives on Earth, not a being that flies on its wings, but forms part of communities like you. Nothing have we omitted from the Book, and they all shall be gathered to their Lord in the End."

In Hadith, the Holy Prophet says : "Surely be kind to the animals; and Allah will reword them for giving them (animals) water; and when they become tired do not make them work." Also the Hadith: "Fear Allah for the sake of these dumb animals."

The love and compassion shown for animals in the religion of Islam points to the fact that the religion does not advocate killing of animals. However, majority of Islam followers are meat-eaters. In fact, majority of meat-eaters across the globe include a high percentage of Christians and Muslims. It will be worthwhile if by going through this book, they understand the deeper meaning of their religious teachings and tilt towards vegetarianism.

3

Vegetarianism is the Natural Way of Life

Human Milk

A man's consumption, when he comes to this world of mortals, begins with milk-human milk. Let us set down to note what is found in milk when analysed carefully. This fluid, Nature's balance of food elements, is made in mother's body for the feeding of a baby, and contains:

Protein	1.5%
Fat	3.5%
Sugar	6.5%
Minerals and salts	0.5%
Water	88.0%

Contents of Mother's Milk

Protein: Is a complex substance found in all living creatures—plants, animals and men. Plants are capable of making their own protein; animals and men are not. So they have to get it in their food. And it is there in the complete food that Nature prepares for the small human creature.

Fat: The creamy substance found in milk is called fat. Fat is useful in many ways to human body. It produces the muscles and tissues; it is a source of warmth and energy; and it repairs and maintains the nerves.

Sugar: Is also present in milk in diluted form. Plants are capable of making sugar out of carbon, hydrogen and oxygen, but men and animals lack this quality, they cannot make sugar of their own. So they need to get is in their food. In so many plants and in all ripe fruits there is sugar. Grains like wheat, rice, maize and oats are very rich in starch and this starch can be changed into sugar in the human digestion.

The minerals and salts in human milk, though so small in amount, are quite essential. As we saw that 88% of the contents of human milk forms of water and minerals and salts are just 0.5%, the smallness of the amount of minerals can be judged or imagined. This 0.5% of minerals and salts figures as follows when analyzed after evaporation of the total water content:

Table 3.1: Mineral and Salts in Human Milk

Mineral	*Percentage (%)*
Sodium	0.003
Calcium	0.006
Magnesium	0.0075
Iron	0.0007
Potassium	0.0012
Phosphorus	0.008
Sulphur	0.0003
Chlorine	0.006
Silicon	0.000007

Other minerals present in human milk include fluorine, iodine, copper, zinc, barium, silica, aluminum and manganese, but in smaller amounts than the above.

If the protein, the fat and the sugar are to be of any use to an infant the above mentioned minerals are also essential. But the first thing to be noticed about the make-up of Nature's food for a baby is the large proportion of water. It shows that food for adults should not be unduly concentrated. So, if we can arrange our meals in a way that we get the necessary sugar or starch, protein, fat and at the same time plenty of water in the food and something approaching the proportions found in human milk, we should be on the right way to a complete food.

Design of Teeth and Suitable Food Variety

As a baby grows, its physical and mental development requires various types of materials at different stages. Teething in a baby is a complex process. Teeth are made mainly of calcium phosphate, and we saw that calcium and phosphorus are two of the minerals found in mother's milk. These minerals are found also in cow's or goat's milk.

The shape of the teeth gives a straight tip as to the sort of food they are designed to deal with. The front teeth are designed for biting into the food and the side teeth for crushing and pulping the food.. We have to use first our front teeth and then our side teeth when eating an apple or a stick of celery.

Thus, keeping in view the design of our teeth we should consume foods that contain a large amount of water and fiber and call our teeth into action. Concentrated foods like dry fruits, nuts, biscuits and chocolate etc. should be consumed in moderate quantity. The more concentrated is the food, the more moderate should be our consumption of it.

Even the shape of "walled-in" oral cavity facilitates the crushing and grinding action of chewing.

The lower jaw has a pronounced horizontal side-to-side motion; the upper and lower molars horizontally slide across one another creating the grinding action of chewing. Accordingly, the molars are not sharp and blade-shaped, but are squared, flat-topped and abut one another forming extended grinding surfaces. The incisors are broad, flattened and spade-shaped and used for cropping and peeling. The canines may be absent, as in cows and sheep; shortened and reduced, as in horses and humans; or dagger-like and used for defense, as in hippos and some primates. Herbivores also usually have carbohydrate digesting enzymes in their saliva that begins the process of digestion while food is still in the mouth. In fact, the purpose of chewing (including chewing the cud) is to mix food with digestive enzymes to facilitate the process of digestion.

As for the carnivore, their, molars are sharp, jagged and blade-shaped. The upper molars vertically slide past the lower molars in a slicing motion when the jaw is closed. These animals do not chew their food. Instead, they slice off huge chunks of meat and swallow them whole. Digestive enzymes which is abundant in herbivore's saliva (to digest the starch in diet) is absent in their's as flesh-digesting (protein, which is a major constituent in flesh diet) enzymes released in the unprotected mouth would quickly destroy the oral cavity.

The Length of the Intestines

The length of human intestine is 10 m.

Plant tissues contain large amounts of fibrous material. The end result is that plant foods require extensive processing to extract their nutritional content. Because of this, herbivores consume smaller, more frequent meals, and tend to have much longer and, in some cases, much more elaborate digestive tracts than their meat-eating counterparts. And Humans are no exception to it.

The human esophagus does not handle poorly chewed food very well. Over 90% of the people who choke to death each year choke on meat.

Only herbivores have an appendix (so does humans!).

No matter how much fat and cholesterol you feed carnivores like dogs and cats, they NEVER develop coronary artery disease

In a typical herbivore, the stomach holds less than 30% of the total capacity of the GI tract. On the other hand, the small intestine is extremely long and is usually more than 10-12 times the body length and has an unlimited capacity or carbohydrate absorption. The large intestine or colon is also relatively long and complex and frequently has a pouched appearance.

Whereas that of a carnivore stomachs are acidic and have huge storage vats that account for 60-70% of the total capacity of their GI tracts. Meat has no fiber and is, therefore, easily digested. Thus, their small intestines are very short (only 3-6 times their body length) and are optimized for protein and fat absorption. Their large intestines are short straight and smooth and designed for evacuation purposes only.

In every respect, humans show the anatomic and physiologic features typical of an herbivore.

Table 3.2 : Carnivores and Herbivores Animals

Carnivores Animals	*Herbivores Animals*
1. Carnivores have sharp pointed teeth and claws with such nails as help them in tearing apart their prey easily.	1. Herbivores have teeth enbedded in flat jaws. Their claws do not have sharp nails but are framed as such to pluck fruits etc. easily.
2. The lower jaws of carnivores move only upward and down-ward and they swallow their food without mastication.	2. The jaws of herbivores can move up ans down left and right, i.e., in all directions. They swallow their food after shewing it.
3. The tongue of meat-eating animal is very rough. They protrude it outnearda to drink water.	3. The tongue of vegetarian animals is quite smooth. They use their lips rather than a protruding tongue to drink.
4. The length of intestines of carnivores is less almost equal to the length of their bodies and about six times the length of their lorso. Due to small intestines they throw out the flesh food before it gets contaminated and poisoned.	4. Harbivores have longer intestines, about four times their body length or twelve times the torso, which can not quickly expel any flesh food.
5. The liver and kidney of meat eating animals are larger in proportion due to which they can throw out the waste material of meat easily.	5. The liver and kidney of vegetarian animals are smaller in proportion and unable to throw out the animal waste easily.

6. The hydrochloric acid content in the digestive system of carnivores is ten times more as compared to that of human beings which digests the meat easily.	6. The hydrochloric acid content vegetarian species is much less and so unable to digest meat easily.
7. The saliva of flesh eaters is acidic.	7. The salive of vegetarian species is alkaline and it contains Ptyaline which is helpful in digesting carbohy-drates.
8. Carnivores have low blood-PH, i.e., it tends to be acidic.	8. Harvivores have higher Blood-PH, i.e., it tends to be on alkaline side.
9. The blood Lipo proteins of the carnivores are different from those of herbivores.	9. In human beings, the Blood-Lipo-Proteins are similar to those of the herbivores.
10. Carnivores have a very strong sense of smell, their eyes glow in the night and their night vision is as good as in the day time. These powers help them in killing their prey.	10. The sense of smell among herbirvores is not so strongly developed and their night vision is nowhere as good as day vision.
11. The sound of meat eating animals is very coarse and frightening.	11. The sound of vegetarian animals is not coarse.
12. The visual power of kids of meat eating animals is almost zero for about a weak after their birth.	12. The offspring of vegetarian animals have normal sight, right from their birth.

The Wholesome Diet

One argument that meat eaters put forward is that vegetarian diet does not provide enough and wholesome nutrition. Let us now see how far this is true.

Sugar

Analysis reveals that fresh ripe fruits, with the exception of bananas and olives, on a general average contain 6% of sugar. Of course some fruits like grapes and some berries have 15-16% of sugar in them, but 6 in the average. Thus, fruits are quite capable of meeting our need of sugar if taken in a planned way. And it is an inconvertible truth that it is quite easy to get all the sugar we need by eating everyday some ripe fruit or a moderate amount of stone-milled flour in the form of bread. The ripe fruit supplies diluted 'living' sugar where as bread supplies starch which our bodies readily convert into sugar. Vegetables like potatoes, carrots and beetroots are also good source of sugar. sugar needs of babies are met by 6.5% of sugar present in mother's milk. The raw juice of sugar-cane contains nearly 19% of sugar.

[(sugar bought from market has 93% of sugar in it—the juice of sugar cane being three times more concentrated than the standard and sugar fifteen times more than required. Taking sugar in high concentration and high quantity is a grave danger to human health. Why so? as this sugar is practically devoid of minerals and vitamins; it ranks as the worst 'deficient food' of modern times. *(a vegetarian diet is no exception to the rule of a balanced diet which should provide all the nutrients in the right quantity and quality and not just excess of one of them)*].

Starch

As for starch, our digestive system very readily converts it into sugar (and this starts in the mouth itself where enzymes in saliva convert starch into simpler sugar), so starch is also a main constituent of our staple food. We saw that human milk does not contain starch, though sugar is present with a good percentage. A growing baby needs starch as it is essential for instant energy to play; an adult needs it to get energy to work. The human digestion is fully and marvelously equipped to digest starch. The saliva—if the food is not swallowed hurriedly—changes the starch into a form of sugar. Later on pancreatic juices and other enzymes complete the process of its metabolism.

Plants are a great source of starch. They build up starch in their normal life-process. They first make sugar from air and water with help of sunlight and then convert it into starch for storage. The only use of this starch we can make is as sugar. The in taken starch is turned back into sugar by our digestive system.

Let us consider the foods that contain starch.

Potato is about 1/5th i.e. 20% starch,

White or brown bread more than half i.e. 50%,

White flour biscuits 2/3rds i.e. 66%,

Corn flour is about 4/5th i.e. 80% starch,

Lentils before cooking have 50% starch,

Oats (raw) also have starch more than 50% and

Polished rice is 80% starch.

So we can rely for our need of starch on any of these starch-foods. Yes, oats, being rich not only in starch but in protein, vitamins and minerals also, and even a little fat, can be chosen for best.

Roughage

Though any roughage is not present in human milk, a baby has regular bowel-motions. It proves that a baby's bowel-muscles act rhythmically without any roughage. But similar is not the case with adults. They have to take a considerable amount of roughage with their staple food. Some of the food items like oat meals (coarse) and whole wheat meal contain considerable amount of roughage. The Oriental people, with whom rice is a staple food, are not afflicted with constipation, though the outer most husks is not included. The rice they consume is cream-coloured and totally different form the polished rice sold in the modern markets of India and the Western countries. This creamy colour rice has a great resemblance with one used in Bihar and West Bengal.

Roughage not only helps in regularizing bowel movements but also adsorbs many harmful chemicals in the food and prevents them from being absorbed in the body.

A non-vegetarian diet is poor source of roughage and many diseases like colon cancer are prevalent in races where non-vegetarian diet is a way of life.

Protein and Vegetarian-Food

Protein is said to be the building block of life. The coding of life is in the form of protein. Proteins are derived from amino acid which are either essential (that is they cannot be synthesized in body) or non-essential (those that can be synthesized by the body from other materials).

Though proteins are majorly building material in the body, when the needs arise, they can be converted into source of energy.

Against a common notion that a vegetarian diet lacks adequate protein for growth and development (from where doe one think that an infant derives its protein-from none other than mothers milk and it is the only thing an infants intestine can handle and provide sufficient nutrition for the fragile early year), a well balanced veg diet is more rewarding than a non-vegetarian diet (and why statistics tell us that uric acid disease is more common in meat eaters).

Plants build up protein with the help of sunlight and water through the process of photosynthesis. Protein circulates in the sap of the plant and in necessary for the formation of chlorophyll. It is packed in concentrated form and generously into the seeds of the plants to make sure that life shall go on.

Seeds like peas, beans, lentils, nut kernel, grains of wheat, barley, maize, rice and other cultivated grasses are very rich in protein.

These are not the only sources of protein available to us but all leaves, roots, stems and fruits, milk of cow, goat and other mammalian animals contain protein in adequate amounts.

As we saw human milk contains 1.5% of protein, cheese has it from 25 to 40 per cent depending on how much water it retains. Let us have a look at the protein content of different vegetarian edibles:

Table 3.3: Protein Content in Different Vegetarian Edibles

Vegetarian Edibles	*Percentage (%)*
Soya flour	43
Wheat germ	35
Peanuts	20
Cheese	25-40
Almond	21
Pinkernels	33
Fresh coconut	4
Fresh peas	5
Raw chestnuts	2
Dried apricots	4
Cooked potatoes	1.5
Bananas	1
Fresh green vegetables average	1

The table shows that vegetables, fruits and grains are very rich in protein and are capable of fulfilling the protein requirement of human body.

[Protein content of red meat and eggs are 25% and 12.5% respectively.]

Fat

Keeping in view the fat contents of human milk which accounts about 3.5% it seems clear that fat is of great importance in our food.

Fats and oils consist of the same three elements as starch and sugar-namely carbon, oxygen and hydrogen. It follows that they, too, are available for combustion. i.e. producing heat and energy (equal amount of fat provide double the energy than carbohydrate). But fat or oil is also used as a protective covering for all cells of the body, muscles and nerves. Thus, fat in food is utilized in two distinct ways—combustion and covering.

A baby needs protection of its tender structure. Though it cannot run and walk, yet every organ needs warmth. Fat provides that adequate insulation as well cushioning as shock absorber for the fragile infantile organs. As the baby grows and becomes active, it's the overall percentage of fat decreases.

Fat again can be of two types saturated as well as unsaturated. About 30% of daily need of nutrients is contained in fats out which 20%is unsaturated and 10% is saturated.

Kernels, apricots, olive, nuts and beans are very rich in fat or oil. Except for chestnuts all the nuts are the richest fat foods available from vegetable kingdom. Soya is unique among beans for its oil content amounting upto 19%. Oil or fat procured from vegetable kingdom contains good per centage of unsaturated fat which is good for human health, while animal fats have high per centage of saturated fat in them which is a great danger to human health causing high blood pressure and heart stroke due to high percentage of cholesterol in them.

Minerals

Human milk contains not only protein, sugar and fat but minerals—both, acid and alkaline. Though the total of these in less than 0.5% (as we saw above), yet they are fully as essential as protein, fat and sugar. The smallness of amount required, is no indication of their lesser importance. Following are the principal alkaline and acid minerals present inhuman milk—Potassium (0.0012%), Sodium (0.003%), Calcium (006%), Magnesium (0.0075), and Iron (0.00007%) are the alkaline whereas phosphorus (0.008%), sulphur (0.001%) silica (0.00007%) and chlorine (0.0060%) are the acid minerals.

The minerals found in milk and other food stuff are mostly in combination; alkalies are usually combined with acids. But the process of digestion and assimilation splits them up to be used for different purposes. Sodium chloride (common salt) is a major ingredient of the clear part of blood, calcium phosphate is a major ingredient of the bones, potassium phosphate and magnesium phosphate is essential to nerve structures.

Apart from these nutritional needs the alkaline minerals are used by the living cells for the vital purpose of clearing out the acid end-products of proteins, starch sugar and fats.

The cells have a profound impulse towards the maintenance of a right balance between acid and alkali in all the fluids and tissues of the body. In the process of nutrition acid in continually and unavoidably formed. There is a continuous flow of acid-wastes coming out from the cells and a steady incoming of alkaline minerals into the cells. Thus, the minerals are essential for conditioning the body.

This need of alkaline and acid minerals can be met easily by fresh water, common salt, fresh raw or ripe fruits and fresh green vegetables. We need not turn towards non-vegetarian foods for these, because non-vegetarian foods one made from dead cells containing high quantity of acid minerals which can be harmful for human health. This is why the alkaline minerals, present in human milk, are considerably higher in amount than that of acid minerals.

And now that the importance of the minerals is very great in our food we should always have in our minds the following table containing the details of the minenals—both acid and alkaline—in the three categories of our food.

Table 3.4: Acid and Alkaline Minerals in our Food

	Principal Alkaline minerals			*Principal Acid minerals*		
	Pot.	*Sod.*	*Cal.*	*Mag.*	*Iron.*	*Phos*
Veg.	264	67	113	12	1.34	33
Fruits	224	2	15.4	14	0.32	19
Grains	6.3	0.75	0.92	2.27	0.17	9.5

The amounts shown are in miligram of every 100 gm of the dried food substance.

Vitamins

Lastly we should not forget the importance of vitamins, lack of which causes many deficiency diseases like rickets, survey, pellagra, beri-beri etc. But we need not worry about the availability of vitamins as they are found in the food stuff we eat daily, except for vitamin "D" which is available in plethora and at no cost in the 'sun' sprouted grains are very rich in rare vitamins like 'E' and 'K'. Butter and vegetable oils one very popular sources of vitamin 'A' (which are usually fortified). We need just to take care of a balanced diet, that too for a balanced vegetarian diet which is natural, whole honest, moral rational, humane and wholesome.

Table 3.5 : Nutrition Contents of Every 100 Gram : Milk and Milk Products

Items	*Proteins*	*Carbo-hydrate*	*Fats*	*Fibre*	*Mine-rals*	*Calo-ries*
Buffalo Milk	4.3	5.0	6.5	-	0.8	117
Cow's Milk	3.2	4.4	4.1	-	0.8	67
Yoghurt	18.3	1.2	20.8	-	2.6	265
Cheese	24.1	6.3	25.1	-	4.2	348
Milk Solids	22.3	25.7	1.6	-	4.3	206
Skimmed Milk Powder	38.0	51.0	0.1	-	6.8	357
Butter	-	-	81.0	-	2.5	729
Ghee	-	-	100.0	-	-	900

Table 3.6 : Nutrition Contents of Every 100 Gram : Meat Products/Eggs

Item	*Proteins*	*Carbo-hydrate*	*Fats*	*Fibre*	*Mine-rals*	*Calo-ries*
Pork	18.7	-	4.4	-	1.0	414
Goat Meat	21.4	-	3.6	-	1.1	118
Mutton Muscles	18.5	-	13.3	-	1.3	194
Fish	8.9 to 76.1	0 to 13.9	0.2 to 19.4		0 to 27.5	59 to 413
Eggs	13.3	-	13.3	-	1.0	173

Table 3.7 : Contents of Every 100 Gram : Plant Products

Items	*Proteins*	*Carbo-hydrate*	*Fats*	*Fibre*	*Minerals*	*Calo-ries*
Buffalo Milk	4.3	5.0	6.5	-	0.8	117
Wheat	12.1	69.4	1.7	1.9	2.7	341
Barley	11.5	69.6	1.3	3.9	1.2	336
Bajra	11.6	67.5	5.0	1.2	2.3	361
Maize	11.1	66.2	3.6	2.7	1.5	342
Grams	17.1	60.9	5.3	3.9	3.0	360
Rice	13.5	48.4	16.2	4.3	6.6	393
Soyabeans	43.2	20.9	19.5	3.7	4.6	432
Rajmah	22.9	60.6	1.3	4.8	3.2	346
Urad	24.0	59.6	1.4	0.9	3.2	347
Lobia	24.1	54.5	1.0	3.8	3.2	323
Moong	24.0	56.7	1.3	4.1	3.5	334
Masoor	25.1	59.0	0.7	0.7	2.1	343
Moth	23.6	56.5	1.1	4.5	3.5	330
Arhar	22.3	57.6	1.7	1.5	3.5	335
Gram Dal	20.8	60.9	5.6	3.9	2.7	360
Ground Nut	26.2	26.7	39.8	3.1	2.5	570
Almonds	20.8	10.5	28.9	1.7	2.9	655
Walnuts	15.6	11.0	64.5	2.6	1.8	687

Contd.

Items	*Proteins*	*Carbo-hydrate*	*Fats*	*Fibre*	*Minerals*	*Calo-ries*
Cashew	21.2	22.3	46.9	1.3	2.4	596
Pista	19.8	16.1	53.5	2.1	2.8	626
Chilgoza	13.9	29.0	49.3	1.0	2.8	615
Kishmish	1.8	74.6	0.3	1.1	2.0	308
Gingelly	18.3	25.0	43.3	2.9	5.2	563
Water Melon Seeds	34.1	4.5	52.6	0.8	3.7	628
Coconut	6.8	18.4	62.3	6.6	1.6	662
Dates	2.5	75.8	0.4	3.9	2.1	317
Munnaqqa	2.7	75.2	0.5	2.2	1.1	316
Amla	0.5	13.7	0.1	3.4	0.5	58
Banana	1.2	27.2	0.3	0.4	0.8	116
Apple	0.2	13.4	0.5	1.0	0.3	59
Cherry	1.1	13.8	0.5	0.4	0.8	64
Grapes	1.0	10.0	0.1	-	0.4	45
Guavas	0.9	11.2	0.3	5.2	0.7	51
Lichi	1.1	13.6	0.2	0.5	0.5	61
Bel Fruit	1.8	31.8	0.3	2.9	1.7	137
Mosambi	0.8	9.3	0.3	0.5	0.7	43
Limes	1.0	11.1	0.9	1.7	0.3	57

Contd.

Items	*Proteins*	*Carbo-hydrate*	*Fats*	*Fibre*	*Minerals*	*Calo-ries*
Orange	0.7	10.9	0.2	0.3	0.3	48
Mulberry	1.1	10.3	0.4	1.1	0.6	49
Phalsa	1.3	14.7	0.9	1.2	1.1	72
Aru	1.2	10.5	0.3	1.2	0.8	50
Papaya	0.6	7.2	0.1	0.8	0.5	32
Mango	0.6	16.9	0.4	0.7	0.4	74
Raspberry	1.0	11.7	0.6	1.0	0.9	56
Water Chestnut	13.4	68.9	0.8	-	3.1	330
Carrot leaves	5.1	13.1	0.5	1.9	2.8	77
Radish leaves	3.8	2.4	0.4	1.0	1.6	28
Bathua leaves	3.7	2.9	0.4	0.8	2.6	30
Methi leaves	4.4	6.0	0.9	1.1	1.5	49
Palak leaves	2.0	2.9	0.7	0.6	1.7	26
Mint	4.8	5.8	0.6	2.0	1.9	48
Cabbage	1.8	4.67	0.1	1.0	0.6	27
Tinda	1.4	3.4	0.2	1.0	0.6	21
Cauliflower	2.6	4.0	0.4	1.2	1.0	30
Ladies Fingers	1.9	6.4	0.2	1.2	0.7	35
Beans	7.4	29.8	1.0	1.9	1.6	158
Potatoes	1.6	22.6	0.1	0.4	0.6	97
Tomatoes	1.5	6.7	0.2	.2	1.2	35

Stay Vegetarian

In the light of above, we can safely pronounce that all the needs of a human body with regard to food consumption, are fulfilled by a vegetarian diet. So, why at all should we kill animals to feed ourselves, many of whom are our pals, servants, mean of recreation and source of joy and comfort? If this simple logic is understood by us, should we not stay vegetarians (who are) or switch over to vegetarianism (who are not.)? And do we need to get into debates of more serious nature like religion, sin, ethics and all that, when this simple logic makes us understand to stick to vegetarian diet?

4

Switching to Vegetarianism

Switching from being a non-vegetarian to become a vegetarian is not as tough an argument as it might seem. It is found that long time flesh-eaters switched to vegetarianism of their own accord without being counseled or forced into it. They voice a variety of reasons from emotional, ethical, and religious to witnessing killing of animals, to effect of media or some other reason. Their experience tells us that they smoothly turned to vegetarianism without looking back or ever tasting flesh again, barring a few. Those who did had an occasional craving for meat in initial years but later on they also forgot all about meat. Let us now go through the voices of such people who take us down their memory lane and let us know how they felt and what were the effects of converting to vegetarian diet on their lifestyle and health, etc.

Reasons for Change

Some people are motivated less by an emotional concern with animal suffering and more by an abstract conviction that animals, along with humans, should be accorded certain rights. They feel that, regardless of whether or not suffering is involved, killing and eating animals is a violation of the animal's most basic right: the right to life. Some people extend their moral philosophy mainly to mammals; others feel that all forms of life have certain rights. These people typically rely less on appeals to emotion than on logical argument to make their point.

Some individuals who view themselves as animal lovers become aware of the inconsistency between caring for animals and eating them. Many who have this experience feel that they are hypocrites. The realization that they are acting in violation of their own values provides a sufficient motivation for these people to change their behaviour. Ben, an accountant, put it this way, "I did it because I just started thinking about where the meat came from. I realized I was a hypocrite, as a supposed animal lover. If I really care about animals, how can I possibly promote an industry based on such terrible cruelty to animals?"

Most people become aware of these issues through contact with the animal welfare movement either through reading animal rights literature or through direct contact with a member of an animal rights organization. Other people decide to join an animal rights organization and adopt vegetarianism at the same time, as part of an over all change in lifestyle. In contrast, some people are active in the animal rights movement for years before they finally make a commitment to stop eating flesh.

Although many ethical vegetarians are influenced by the animal rights movement, others come to the conclusion that eating animals is wrong on their own. In some cases, for a period of time a person thinks that he or she is the only person in the world who doesn't eat animals for moral reasons. For these individuals, discovering that other ethical vegetarians exist comes as a surprise and a relief.

A few people are led to ethical vegetarianism through working with animals.

Once people are convinced that killing and eating animals is wrong, their consciences and their need to think of themselves as responsible people, require that they live as vegetarians. It is an orientation to one's diet that is relatively demanding. Because refraining from meat is a moral imperative, lapses generate feelings of guilt remorse. Consequently, ethical vegetarians are less likely than those motivated by other concerns to revert back to meat-eating either temporarily or permanently.

Concern Over Health

A concern over health is another major reason for abstaining from meat. Health vegetarians can be divided into two groups: those who are primarily concerned with food additives, and those who are primarily concerned with the role of meat and animal fat in various degenerative diseases.

Those in the first group adopt a vegetarian diet, not so much because of the meat itself, but because of the antibiotics, growth hormones, and stimulants given to farm animals, as well as the chemicals used to treat and preserve meats. People concerned about the additives fond in meat typically try to avoid all processed foods that contain artificial ingredients and preservatives.

A group of health vegetarians are those concerned about the implications of a diet containing high levels of animal fat for heart disease, cancer, and other health disorders. A number of people in this group work in the medical professions. As such, they are familiar with the recent medical literature linking diet to a variety of degenerative diseases.

Some health vegetarians are completely unaware of the medical literature showing a correlation between meat-centered diets and various diseases. Instead, they discover through personal experience that they feel better and are generally healthier when not eating meat. These people typically start off adopting a vegetarian diet for a period of time as an experiment; later, when they find they like the outcome, their commitment to vegetarianism is established. Roy was traveling around the country with no destination and a pocketful of money when he had the following experiences; "I started paying attention to how I felt after eating certain types of food. I noticed that when I ate meat, my body felt heavy and dull, and that when I ate vegetarian meals, my body usually felt good. Later I did a lot of reading on nutrition, and I experimented with different types of diets. I decided that I was definitely healthier as a vegetarian."

The notion that a meatless diet is health-promoting is consistent with their medical research. It is also supported by the many personal accounts we heard from health vegetarians. Some told us that they had suffered from health problems for years and had turned to vegetarianism as a way of dealing with them. We have describe some of these cases in detail later when we discuss the personal implications of a meatless diet. It is worth pointing out here, however, that for these people, a change in diet (often accompanied by other changes in lifestyle, such as in-creased exercise) resulted in major and dramatic improvements in health, and this became a powerful motive for their continuing to live as vegetarians.

Specific Experiences

An anthropologist once told us a story about an experience she had while living in an island society. The traditional diet on this Island society consisted of plant foods and fish, but in recent years frozen mutton had been imported from Australia. One day a group of children asked her what this meat was, assuming it must have been some sort of fish. When she explained that it was an animal and showed them a picture of sheep, the children were horrified. To them the thought of eating an animal that had fur was disgusting.

Many vegetarians would agree with the children in this story. And often meat-eaters often admit to feeling a fit squeamish when reminded that they regularly eat the bodies of dead animals. But most of the time people do a good job of "forgetting" where meat comes from.

Sometimes, however, individuals have experiences that force this knowledge out of the backs of their minds and into their full awareness. As a result, they are led to reexamine their eating habits, and eventually to give up meat. The particular experiences that produce this outcome are diverse. In our sample, the types of experiences and the percentage of people reporting them, a direct insight into the nature of meat (10%), seeing food animals being transported (4%), witnessing animals being killed (3%), practicing meditation or yoga (4%), dissecting animals in a classroom (2%) and having a major illness (1%).

Insight into the Nature of Meat

A feeling of revulsion, brought on by a sudden insight into what meat is and where it comes from, is the most commonly mentioned experience. Typically this recurs when people are eating or about to eat. Judging from people's accounts, these 'meat insight' experiences have an immediate impact on behaviour.

"I stopped eating meat seven years ago abruptly when I took a bite out of a piece barbecued chicken and found a vein sticking out half eaten." The expression, "A few days before I became vegetarian, I came home from school and there was left over roast in a pan. I saw the bone—it was a hip. And I began to think, "what am I doing? I am eating a corpse." The whole thing became repulsive to me and I developed a dislike for meat right then. I had been eating tongue when I saw a cow in my mind's eye. The cow was whole, I couldn't finish the food. I quit eating all flesh."

Meat insight experiences are extremely powerful, and people often describe them in strong terms. As one person said, "It was as if a great light came on in my mind and I could suddenly see flesh eating for what it really is—barbaric, horrible and disgusting". These moments of insight can lead to a complete reevaluation of one's eating habits; many people become "aesthetic" vegetarians shortly afterward. As Sukhbinder put it "The moment I realized that I was eating the furry creatures I loved, I refused to eat meat again."

In a few cases, people are confronted with the reality of flesh-eating when some one makes a joke at mealtime about meat being a dead animal. The realization that it's not really a joke means that for the soon-to-be vegetarian, eating meat is no laughing matter.

I was 12 when I stopped eating meat. I didn't like it, my friend stuck a fork into a leg of lamb and said "Baaa, Baaa" I quit eating all flesh after that.

At an evening meal of homemade soup my sister joked to me, "There is a dead cow in your soup" I looked at the beef and decided that I did not want to eat dead cows.

I came home after class and one of my room-mates said, "There is some meat in the refrigerator if you want to make a sandwich. "I looked inside and there on plate was a sheep fetus—my room-mate's biology project. It seemed funny at the time in a macabre just of way, but I thought about that foetus the next few times I ate meat.

Meat insight experience sometimes can also occur when preparing or cooking meat. On these occasions, the sight, smell or feel of raw meat causes people to associate it with a formerly living animal. An odd juxtaposition of events provided Kalim, a home maker, with an insight into what she was about to eat. Although it ruined her Thanksgiving dinner, the outcome, as far as he was concerned, was for the best.

My wife and I were always animal lovers but for many years did not make the connection between what was on our platter and what was in our hearts. One thanksgiving I had to wash a turkey in the bathtub because of its size. The realization that its body was just like my dog that I washed in the same tub was overwhelming. We became vegetarian that night.

Food insight experiences sometimes have unusual origins. One woman told us about a nightmare she had about eating meat. The day before, she had bought some meat from a butcher shop, and the sound of hacking while she was standing in line made an impression on her. That night she had a nightmare about a cow being sliced up and served while still alive. The next day she became a vegetarian. In her case she had been uncomfortable with the idea of eating animals for some time, the nightmares was simply a reflection of her growing anxiety over eating flesh.

Another unusual story comes from a mother who became a vegetarian after having to explain the origin of meat to her young daughter. Being forced to confront the truth led her to perceive the chicken on her plate, not as her dinner, but as a dead animal.

My family was sitting down to a meal of fried chicken and my young daughter brought her toy chicken to the table with her. My husband's aunt said, "Eat your chicken". My daughter seemed surprised at these words. She looked at her aunt, her toy chicken and then at her plate. At that moment I realized that I would have to explain to my child where meat comes from. How could I tell this innocent child who loved animals so dearly that her own mother and father actually fed on slaughtered cows, pigs and chickens. All at once the sight of the dead chicken on by plate nauseated me. I realized that I was deeply ashamed of the fact that I ate meat. I knew the only answer was for me to become vegetarian and to raise my daughter as one as well.

Some of the saddest stories we heard were from people who, as children, had their pets dished up for dinner. As one person said, "I first seriously decided to do without meat when my mother cooked my pet rabbit in a stew and I ate it without knowing it". Another person came home from school one day, looked in the refrigerator, and saw a rabbit sliced up on a plate. She asked her mother, "Is this my rabbit?" It was. Surely nothing can drive home more clearly to children the connection between the meat on their plates and a living animal than to see their own pets cooked and served.

It is curious that meat insight experiences are not more common than they are. Many people, for example, handle meat everyday when cooking; yet the sight and smell of blood repulse them. Perhaps individuals who are disgusted by meat simply have "weak" stomachs. However, this seems unlikely. Many people who touch meat (which is muscle tissue and fat) without qualms would feel queasy about manipulating the intestines, brains, or eyes of the same animal. And handling the flesh of a dog etc would probably disgust many people in India even though these animals are considered food sources in other parts of the world. Even internal organs such as beef tongue, tripe, oxtail and brains are eaten only by a minority of people.

These observations reflect the fact that humans 'compartmentalize' their thinking. This allows animals defined as food and those not defined as food to be perceived differently. Psychologists are aware that people use a variety of defenses and rationalization to protect them selves from the unpleasant implications of their behaviour. In the case of meat-eating, people use denial to convince themselves that beaf, meat, pork, chicken and lamb are not really the body of animals. People also have an almost magical belief that cooking transforms raw flesh from something that is completely unpalatable into something that is edible—as if the application of heat transforms the body of an animal into a steak, a hamburger, or a drumstick. In spite of the current penchant for Sushi, most people would cringe at the prospect of eating a raw pot roast.

These tendencies are reinforced by advertising and the meat industry. For example, old fashioned butcher shops once posted pictures of steers with dotted lines superimposed on their bodies delineating the various cuts of meat, with images of roasts, steaks, and ribs decorating the borders. However marketing studies revealed that these charts were offensive to many shoppers; people did not want to be reminded that they were eating animals. Consequently these images are rarely seen in the meat sections of modern supermarkets.

Witnessing the Killing of Animals

Similar to meat insight experiences are occasions on which people witness the slaughtering of animals. Some individuals are so upset after seeing animals being killed that they stop eating meat on the spot. In some cases, this experience occurs during childhood. For example, the following woman, now 35, became vegetarian when she was five years old.

I was visiting my grandparents on the farm. I remember being real upset by it. I saw the whole process from the animal being alive and petting it to then seeing it butchered. I have vague memories of it now, but I remember it happening and refusing to have anything to do with eating animals after that. People who are raised on farms have a good deal of exposure to farm animals. Having the opportunity to experience an emotional bond with an animal, only to see it later sent to slaughter, can result in a strong predisposition to vegetarianism later in life. Rajinder Kaur, a dietician, recounted a particularly painful experience from the past:

I was raised on a farm and did not like killing chickens from an early age. I exhibited a champion Black-Angus 4-H calf who cried when I left it. Actually we both cried. I knew then that he knew what was in store for him. I didn't eat meat for a long time after that.

The above accounts suggest that children are especially sensitive to the killing of animals. Perhaps it is because they, unlike adults, have not yet been strongly conditioned into believing that slaughtering and eating animals is normal and appropriate. Over time the ability of most children to empathic with animals becomes blunted by a culture that treats animals largely as objects to be used.

The sight of animals being slaughtered can be just as upsetting for adult as it is for children. A visit to a slaughter house, in particular, is a grim experience that can make a vegetarian out of the hardiest meat-eater. The following woman visited a slaughterhouse to find out for herself what happens:

I decided to take a visit to one of the abattoirs just down the road where I lived at that time. The smell of blood and fear made me so ill that I had to cut my visit short. I went out to the car and threw up and cried for ages. I have not eaten meat since that day.

If people who visit the abattoir feel this disgusted, what would have been of those who work in abattoir? First there is probably self selection occurring, such that workers who are sensitive to the suffering of animals quit after a short time and find employment elsewhere. Secondly, after working in a slaughterhouse for a period of time, most people become emotionally desensitized. Although the first few hours and days might be difficult, after witnessing thousands of animals being killed, even a sympathetic person would exhibit little emotional reaction. Nevertheless we encountered a couple of ex-slaughterhouse workers who later become vegetarians, so not everyone is able to habituate to the daily carnage.

Given the emotional impact of visiting a slaughter house, it seems likely that many people would become vegetarian if animals were killed and processed in supermarket parking lots instead of behind closed doors in remote country areas. For some people however witnessing the slaughter of animals is not necessary; merely the sight of animals being transported to slaughterhouse—a common experience in rural areas—is the final straw. One respondent had already taken the first tentative steps toward giving up meat when he had an unsettling experience. As he said, "During a car ride following a cattle truck, a cow looked straight into my eyes, and I was certain it knew that it was going to its death." After that he became a vegetarian.

Two individuals in our sample were influenced by the killing of companion animals. One man, a university student, worked for a time as a veterinarian's assistant and had the unpleasant duty of euthanizing animals. Similarly, a woman who managed an animal shelter became concerned about the "massive killing of healthy pets ex-pets." For her, "vegetarianism helps to compensate for all the animals I must kill as part of my job".

Dissections in Biology Classroom

Classroom experiments on organisms compel many people to consider vegetarianism. Although biology class dissections often desensitize students to the needs of animals or to their ability to experience pain, the opposite also occurs in the following story:

I became a vegetarian when I was a sophomore in high school. I was motivated to do so by a biology class project where I had to dissect a fetal pig. The pigs that the class dissected had been taken from their mother's womb when their mothers had been slaughtered. This project made me realize the cruelty of killing animals for food.

Experience of Operation Theatre

The most unexpected experience perhaps was that of two people who became vegetarians after experiencing pain and contemplating their own mortality, led to a new sympathy for the plight of animals. Abdul Ansari told us that after an operation for cervical cancer, he came to realize "how precious all life is" John, a Keralite told us his story:

Four years ago I went to hospital for an operation on polyps in my bladder. I went through terrible, agonizing spasms of pain. I came out of hospital and for a year or more thought about the terrible pain. I got to think about animals. I got to realize that millions of animals were suffering that same terrible pain that I had felt. So I went vegetarian.

Associations

Some people become vegetarians through their involvement in groups or associations that require or recommend vegetarianism. The two major types of organizations represented in our sample are animal rights organizations mentioned by 10 % of all respondents) and religious groups (mentioned by 7% of respondents). Religious groups with vegetarian elements include the Seventh Day Adventists, the International Society for Krishna Consciousness, and follower of Sri Chinmoy or other religious teachers. In most cases people are attracted to the group of religious teachers. In most cases people are attracted to the group for religious reasons and adopt vegetarianism shortly after joining.

In recent years, animal welfare organizations have been directing more of their attention to issues involving farm animals. This change in emphasis has led many to encourage their members to practice vegetarianism. Consequently many individuals give up met shortly after joining one of these groups. However, for some people, particularly those who have been involved in animal welfare activities for a long time, the relation between compassion for animals and vegetarians takes many years to "sink in". These contrasting lengths of time are illustrated in the following two quotations:

> "I became involved in the animal welfare movement and immediately saw a conflict between saving cats and killing cows. I read a flyer that stated if I ate chicken twice a week, I was guilty of killing that chicken. At that instant, my consciousness changed and I knew that I was not capable of harming or killing an animal just for its flesh and couldn't justify having someone else do it for me. I had been actively and profoundly involved in animal welfare work for approximately twenty years. It suddenly occurred to me one day that eating habits and my animal-related activities were incongruous. I began to question how I would fight so hard to protect animals with one hand and stick a knife and fork in them with the other."

As the above quotations suggest, a belief in animal welfare alone is often insufficient to get people to stop eating meat. For many, a little extra motivation is necessary. Some animal rights supporters experience pressure from others in the movement to become vegetarian. This pressure sometimes subtle and sometimes strong and direct—leads many to bring their eating habits in line with their ideologies.

Occasionally, however pressure from people outside the movement does the trick. A typical situation is one in which, during an argument over animal rights, animal advocates are confronted with the inconsistency between their beliefs and their meat-eating vegetarians, the realization that their opponents are correct is a strong incentive for these people to take the first step toward vegetarianism. Abdulla, for example, had a disagreement with his boss, a doctor about the use of animals in medical experiments. During their discussion, he pointed out the conflict between his professed interest in animal rights and his diet. His comments led him to realize that he was indeed acting inconsistently in treating food-animals differently from other animals. Today, Abdulla is an ethical vegan. As he said, "I am glad he pointed it out to me."

Effect of Films

Sometimes a film or video is responsible for a change to vegetarianism. Occasionally, the influence of films is very indirect. For example, after watching the "Kung Fu" TV series, Ray became interested in Zen Buddhism and through that vegetarianism. In most cases, however, the impact of a film is immediate, particularly if the film depicts animal suffering or slaughter. Some people, for example, become upset after watching films about the food or fur industries on television. These films, it seems, can be educational on a moral as well as factual level.

When I was 13 years old I saw a programme on TV on the harp seal slaughter. I shall never forget seeing the seal pup as it was clubbed to death, and the way the mother followed the hunters as they dragged the carcass along the ice. I have never eaten, nor used animal products since.

Other people are strongly influenced by films with a specific vegetarian message, such as vegetarian world, narrated by William Shatner, and the 'The Animal Film', (a film about the treatment of animals by the meat, cosmetics, and medical research industries). Some people mention watching videos on vegetarianism after enjoying a meatless meal at Govinda's-restaurants which are run by the International Society for Krishna Consciousness.

Although mentioned less often than other sources, films can have a powerful impact when viewed under the right circumstances. The power of film derives from the sense of immediacy and reality conveyed by the visual image. Clearly it is one thing to read about animal suffering, and something else to see it. The following story from Harjit Chadha, vegetarian and freelance writer, illustrates the power of visual images to change opinions.

Hearing that The Animal Film, a documentary depicting various ways in which humans abuse and exploit non-humans, including graphic footage of factory farming and animals being slaughtered, was going to be aired on our local public station, I told my parents of it and asked them if they would please try to watch it, knowing that they couldn't probably handle watching the whole thing, but hoping that they might watch even a bit of it. They did watch all of it, to my surprise. My mother told me that it had upset my father greatly for many days afterward. He is in his sixties, as is my mother; both have eaten meat all their lives. My previous efforts to talk to them about vegetarianism, and to be an example of a happy, healthy, well-adjusted person who chooses not to eat meat, had been met with indifference and even some skepticism on my father's part. But to make along story shorter, my mother next informed me after we had been to the supermarket that my father had decreed that he would have no more meat in his house, nor would he eat anywhere else. So this wonderful film helped to make two new ethical vegetarians. It was one of the happiest days of my life.

Aesthetic Reasons

Another group of vegetarians give up flesh for "aesthetic" reasons; that is, they feel that meat is unappealing, unappetizing, or downright repulsive. Many people in this group say they avoid flesh because they do not like its flavor or texture. In some cases, people have felt this way since childhood, and consequently, have never been big meat-eaters. For these people, becoming vegetarian is simply a matter of following their natural preferences.

Some people develop an aversion to animal flesh later in life. Sometimes this change is linked to a specific experience, such as visiting a slaughterhouse. More often a dislike of meat is linked to a gradually evolving awareness of what meat really is. People who think clearly about where the steaks on their plates come from cannot escape the fact that meat is nothing more than the muscle, issue, fat, veins, and blood of a dead animal. Once people fully realize what they are eating, many find it impossible to dine on meat a hearty appetite. For these individuals, Vegetarianism is the next step.

On the positive side, some people enjoy being vegetarian because vegetarian food is delicious and tastes better than meat. As Sharon put it, "Part of what sold me, was how delicious vegetarian cuisine actually is." Often these people start off, like many others, expecting meatless meals to be tasteless and baring. A few encounters with well-prepared vegetarian food at restaurants or friend's homes however, convince them that they can derive considerable gastronomic pleasure living as vegetarians.

Personal Growth as a Reason

Personal growth vegetarians place their primary emphasis on self development. They recognize that abstaining from animal flesh confers many benefits, including improvements in health, spirituality, and a sense of moral purpose. The particular benefits themselves, however, are less important than the fact that vegetarianism helps them to grow and to achieve their full potential. As George, a physics graduate student, said, "I want to be the best that I can be, so I decided that I should be vegetarian."

Many people in this group spend years trying out different philosophies. Some describe themselves as "Searchers" or "Seekers." In most cases, vegetarianism is adopted as a component of a larger and continuing process of self-growth. For a few, vegetarianism occupies a central role as the key element in their personal development.

Some adopt a vegetarian diet as a way of correcting some perceived fault in their characters. These people might be described as "Vegetarian Puritans." For example, Mark stopped eating meat to refine his sexual urges and make them less "bestial." Another individual felt that meat-eating was a form of gluttony: a self-indulgent and unnecessary gratification of the senses. As such meat-eating was a weakness to be overcome: "I had sorrow and suffering due to my gluttony. I was suffering from psychic pain caused by over nutrition. I used to be addicted to meat excesses as a true sensualist. So, in order to subordinate my appetite to my weak will power, I decided to adopt complete vegetarianism.

Hence vegetarianism becomes a way of self control and self realization in many.

Yoga and Meditation

The experiences that impel most people to give up meat-eating are unpleasant. In contrast meditation and yoga provide attractive and enjoyable routes to vegetarianism for a few people. Practitioners of these disciplines often say that a meatless diet is a natural and inevitable step. Many claim that the adoption of a vegetarian diet under these circumstances is effortless and "just seems to happen".

I was taking a yoga class and it felt perfect to me. I eagerly practiced the exercises on my own as well as in class. Slowly the desire to eat meat and put harmful substances into my body vanished. It was easy.

Why should people doing yoga and meditation lose their desire to eat flesh? Most likely, this is due to the fact that these practices require people to spend a good deal of time attending closely to their bodies. With their attention focused on how they are feeling, they realize that a meal based on flesh and animal fat often leaves them feeling sluggish. This is because animal products take longer time to digest than do fruits, vegetables and other plant foods. And to the extent that well balanced vegetarian meals led to improvements in energy and mood, the desire to enhance one's well-being through a good diet should be reinforced.

Other Reasons

(i) *World Hunger :* Some people become vegetarian because they see meat consumption in the West as being partly responsible for world hunger. These individuals are aware of the wastefulness of livestock production as a source of food. As we pointed out earlier, a larger number of people can be supported by using a given area of land to grow crops directly for human consumption than by using the land to grow crops to feed livestock.

- It takes an average of 2,500 gallons of water to produce a single pound of meat. According to Newsweek, "The water that goes into a 1,000 pound steer could float a destroyer." In contrast, it takes only 25 gallons of water to produce one pound of wheat.

- These individuals believe that becoming vegetarians is one small but necessary step in decreasing the demand for meat in the West, and hence, in the eventual freeing of land for producing crops this could be used to feed the poor. Even this small act gives people a sense that they have done something useful and positive. As Roberta said, "I figured we can't change the world, but i can contribute a little bit toward eliminating world hunger."

For many, abstaining from meat is a symbolic gesture of solidarity with hungry people around the world. At the same time, it also represents a rejection of the wasteful practices, and the mixed up values of our own society.

Millie and Bob are examples of vegetarians who are concerned about world hunger. Together they operate a farm in Maine designed to serve as a model of self-sufficiency in food production. They are also involved in investigating new techniques of forestry and energy production that are environmentally sound. As they told us, "We became vegetarians because of land use. It's wasteful of land to be meat and animal product eaters. Becoming farmers has made it all much more understandable."

(ii) *Non-violence :* Many vegetarians do not distinguish between the killing of animals and the killing of humans. Accordingly, they see a link between their diets and issues of peace and non-violence. For some, this link is a very personal one, whereas for others it has society-wide implications.

At the personal level, some vegetarians adopt a philosophy of harmlessness toward all living things. For these people to eat meat is to participate in a deplorable act of violence—even murder. They believe that as vegetarians, they are eliminating an unwanted and unnecessary source of violence from their lives.

On a broader level, rejecting all forms of violence in one's own life may have a beneficial effect on the larger society. Some individuals believe that adopting a non-violent vegetarian diet is a small but positive step for world peace. Often, these people work or have worked in the peace movement. Over time, they have come to feel that it is hypocritical to work for world peace and, at the same time, dine on the bodies of slaughtered animals. Many believe that by living as vegetarians, they set a positive example of non-violence for others and become more effective in advocating the cause of peace. To be a true pacifist, some argue, one must be a vegetarian. Marilyn a masseuse, put it this way:

> "It's something like a non-violence pledge. I wanted to take on a non-violent lifestyle, and I figured that to get rid of violence in the world you can begin with what you're eating."

We have already discussed non-violence as a reason for vegetarianism in diffrenet religions of the world.

While talking of non-violence it will be injudicious not to mention Mahatma Gandhi who led was an ardent follower and preacher of vegetarianism.

(iii) *Vegetarianism, a Natural way of life:* Some vegetarians believe that humans are designed to be plant-eaters and, correspondingly, that meat-eating is unnatural for our species. As supporting evidence, they point out that our physical make up is more akin to that of herbivores than to carnivores. For example, carnivores, unlike humans, have sharp teeth for cutting through skin and bone; humans, like herbivores, have broad molars designed to grind plant foods. Carnivores, unlike humans, can run fast and have sharp claws for catching their prey; humans, on the other hand, are incapable of outrunning and catching an animal such as a deer or rabbit. And carnivores, unlike humans, have strong digestive acids and short intestines to excrete decaying animal matter quickly. Humans, like herbivores, have weak digestive acids and long intestines which are necessary for the slow digestion of plant foods. Many vegetarian believe that humans become "sidetracked" from their original diet.

Most "natural vegetarians" try to simplify their lives. They avoid accumulating material objects, recycle wastes when possible and minimize their consumption of energy from fossil fuels. They prefer to spend their leisure time outdoors in rural areas and avoid the nightlife available in big cities. To them, vegetarianism is another change they have made on the way toward a simpler, more harmonious way of life.

Johan, who works at a food store, is a vegetarian because it is "more natural" than eating meat. He publishes his own natural foods newsletter has few possessions, dresses simply and spends as much time outdoors as possible.

In the opinion of a clerk, the ideal world is one in which all things are left as untouched as possible. As he says, "I like things in their natural order, the way the universe intended". Others like him, feel that human should not try to dominate and change the natural world, and that our present attitudes and behaviour are likely to result in an ecological disaster. Nothing is more unnatural than keeping animals in captivity in modern factory farms. Not only are their meat and milk unsuited for human consumption but keeping animals penned up and unable to roam freely is a violation of their natural inclinations.

Social Influence/Conformity

A few people stop eating meat primarily for social reasons. This typically occurs because they are living with people who are vegetarian. Under these circumstances, it is easier, and more fun, to become vegetarian as well. In one case, this came about when the person was living for a period of time with a family of vegetarian. She discovered that she enjoyed the diet and decided to stick to it when she later moved out. Another person adopted the diet during his college days after his room-mates all gave up eating meat. Although relatively rare in our sample, as vegetarianism becomes more widespread, the number of people who give up eating meat for primarily social reasons will undoubtedly increase.

A small number of people have motives for giving up flesh that are idiosyncratic and difficult to classify. For example, one person became vegetarian for a change of pace; "The basic reason for changing my diet was boredom. I was just really tired of my diet and wanted a change. The more I learned, and the more involved I got, the more I liked it. It was fun and a new learning experience."

One person took it as a challenge, just to see if she could do if;

"Really I did it just for the challenge of it whenever you challenge yourself—like fasting for a couple of days—you are also challenging yourself mentally. That was also part of the reason—to see how long I could do it."

For another person, vegetarianism was a way of setting herself apart from a society with which she largely disagreed; "When I grew up and left school at 16, I looked around the world and realized what a wicked place it was and how dishonest, cruel, and underhanded most people were. I embraced vegetarianism eagerly but not for altruistic reasons. I wanted to be different because I did not want to be party to the ways by the world with its cruelties, stupid religions, and so on. By becoming vegetarian, I would be seen to be different in not uncertain manner.

A couple of people said they had no particular reason for becoming vegetarian; it just seemed like a good idea at the time. Clearly, these people are casual in their approach to life. In contrast, Jim had a complex philosophical position worked out; "The primary reason was and is the desire not to be a predator. I figured that as long as my ultimate identity and purpose as well as the true nature of this place were unknown. I would be philosophically dishonest in killing animals just to maintain my own presence in this possibly meaningless parade of life and death. This does not imply that I assume it is wrong to kill animals and eat them. It seems that whoever created this ecosystem in which we find ourselves designed some animals to eat other animals. We are fully a party of this system, but we have the option of choosing to go with either the consumer-consumer battle for survival, or to take a mellower route. Either is legitimate. I believe those people who go hunting for deer or birds or go fishing and then eat what they kill are not doing anything wrong. But I want to take a different course."

Vegetarians mention a variety of people who influenced their decisions to stop eating flesh. The largest group consists of friends (mentioned by 17% of all vegetarians) followed by casual acquaintances (7%); parents (4%); spouses (3%); children (3%); teacher, doctor or other professionals (3%); extended family (2%); and siblings (1%). How do these people get the message across. In most cases, vegetarian friends and family members actively, but gently, encourage the change. This encouragement usually consists of a basic exposure to the idea, along with dissuasion, as the following quotations illustrate; "I did it gradually because my Dad was health conscious and he would go to health food places. We did not care for it that much, but once in a while we would go with him. I went gradually from there.

I grew up in an orphanage with 50 children. One of our nurses was vegetarian and she used to take me her room and make little salads and talk to me about how cruel it is to kill animals. She convinced me and I have been a vegetarian since I was 11, 52 years ago."

Some individuals stop eating meat after people they are living with—either room-mates or family members—become vegetarian. In some cases, people willing follow suit because they are impressed by the example set by the new vegetarian in their midst. In other cases, they change simply because it is more convenient to maintain a completely meatless household. As several people pointed out, cooking two separate meals every day quickly becomes an unnecessary chore. In a few cases, people have little choice; it comes down to a decision between giving up meat or moving out. As Vikram Singh, a university student from Chandigarh said, "I was persuaded by my room-mate to become a vegetarian. If I hadn't they would have kicked me out of the house.

Occasionally, the first person in a household to change is a child rather than an adult. When children decide to become vegetarians, parents generally do everything they can to force them to eat meat again. Usually parental pressure wins out and the vegetarian experiment is short lived. But there are exceptions. The following story from Balbir Singh, a homemaker illustrates how a shift in family eating habit was initiated by her eight-year old daughter, "One day we were eating a Sunday lunch-lamb-when my daughter suddenly asked, "what was this meat before you cooked it? I told her it was a lamb, and she announced that she would not eat because she liked lambs. She was eight and a half years old. I thought it was time to discuss vegetarianism with her. I tried to give her a balanced view but she said she no longer would eat meat. When I started cooking stuff for my daughter, I also started to eat a share of it. A year later, I decided I didn't like the idea of killing animals. So I joined my daughter in vegetarianism."

Another frequently occurring situation is for people to have their first exposure to vegetarianism while traveling with or visiting vegetarian friends or family members. After trying it for a while, these people discover they enjoy meatless cuisine and the change becomes permanent. Gurmeet, a business consultant, had his first exposure to meatless meals when his cousin came to visit and did a good deal of vegetarian cooking.

As he said, "I thought it was silly at first, but it sparked my awareness.

Although friend and family are common influences, new acquaintances can also serve as catalysts. Some people find their curiosity is aroused after a change encounter with a vegetarian. For example, Kalim, a retired teacher and her daughter were on a backpacking trip in Kaziranga National Park when they met a young vegetarian couple. A conversation on the merits of a meatless diet started them thinking, and later they decided to decrease their own meat consumption. That was 10 years ago; today Kalim, aged 70 is a semi-vegetarian.

A transitory meeting with a vegetarian seems unlikely to change something as fundamental as someone's diet.But this is precisely what happens to many people. How is such influence possible. In many cases meeting a vegetarian for the first time shatters a central belief; that it is necessary to eat meat in order to like. Correspondingly it triggers the insight that it is possible to survive in good health and in good spirits on a plant-centered diet. The following story illustrates the narrow conception many people hold about food and diet. Nirbhay, a lacto-ovo-vegetarian for 15 years, first came to reevaluate his own beliefs after meeting a member of a society where vegetarianism is common.

I met a man from Sri Lanka who had never eaten meat in his life, nor had hardly anyone on his island. As if it just wasn't part of their culture. This made me realize that a core assumption with which I had been programmed all along—that one has to eat animals to live, and if you don't you wither away and die—was obviously false, as this person had lived all his life without ever taking a bite of an animal. I think the first hand proof pushed me into making my first move towards a flesh free diet.

On other occasions, people are impressed by the health and attractiveness of vegetarians they meet. Some people react favorably when they are introduced to young vegetarians who are fit, muscular and athletic. Others are surprised to meet elderly vegetarians who have the appearance and behaviour of people many years younger. Julie, a beautician, had been told that a vegetarian diet might improve her hypoglycemia, but she had serious doubts about the possibility of remaining healthy without eating meat. However, she was later convinced of the soundness of a fleshless diet after an encounter with an elderly vegetarian, "I met this 83-year old woman who was vegetarian. I had never been exposed to it, and I thought it was easy. But when I met this woman I was totally impressed—she had a lot of energy and vitality. She still had three businesses that she was running. Plus she had a lot of young male friends knocking on her door wanting to be in her company because of her vitality."

Sometimes the influence of other people operates in unexpected ways. For example, Begum, a primary school teacher was persuaded to become vegetarian by, if all people, her butcher, "I used to buy for Rs. 150 sides of beef and lots of chicken. Then the delivery man told me of seeing cows being killed and how some died slowly and how it almost made him not want to be a butcher. It put me off buying sides of beef. The occasional tuft of lamb's wool on the meat made me feel sad but I had been brought up in a minister's family where we were taught that all meat is OK to eat. However, I new had doubts because of the butcher, and I stopped eating meat."

All in all, our research shows that vegetarianism often grows through process of personal influence, passing from friend to friend, from family member to family member and from acquaintance to acquaintance. This influence can take the form of direct persuasion, but it more often takes the form of information, mild encouragement, and the provision of an attractive role model. The fact that many people are influenced in such subtle ways indicates that one can bring about a good deal of change in the behaviours of others simply by living as a vegetarian. Many vegetarians are probably having more influence on the people around them and they realize.

Influence of Literature/Information

Many people claim that printed matter was instrumental in their decisions to become vegetarian. Books are mentioned most often (by 25% of all respondents), followed by newsletters (7%) magazine or newspaper articles (4%), animal rights leaflets (2%) and academic journals (1%). Of those who mention books, three-fourth refers to animal rights and animal welfare literature and one half mention Peter Singer's work, *Animal Liberation*—the single most commonly mentioned book we encountered.

Balbir, who is active in the animal liberation movement in Punjab, was strongly influenced by Singer's book. His story reflects the fact that reaching about the treatment of animals can be unpleasant, and for this reason, is often avoided. The emotional impact of this material, however, is undoubtedly a strong motivator of behaviour change, "It'd happened upon an illustrated review of Professor Peter Singer's book, *Animal Liberation*. I read the review, rushed out and bought the book, and promptly put it to rest in the book case. It was too difficult and distressing to confront. One day, a year later, I pulled up behind a truck load of pigs, obviously abattoir-bound. That clinched it. I knew that they, or others like them, would be on my plate that night. Back home, I pounced on Singer's book, read every word, and knew that I had become vegetarian."

Some ethical vegetarians also mention Town Regan's book, *The Case for Animal Rights*, as having been influential. Because Regan's work is more academic in tone than Singer's, it tends to be of particular interest to those who have had some exposure to university level philosophy courses. Sarah received more than a good grade in her university course after becoming familiar with Regan's book. She said, "In 1986, I took a philosophy class that really got me started. For my class paper I decided to write on 'Man's Treatment of Animals'. I was having trouble finding information on the subject. Sooner or later I came across Tom Regan's book, *The Case for Animal Rights*. My term paper was a success all 27 pages of it. Before I received my grade I had given up all meat and poultry but not fish. I soon read other books on vegetarianism, and I knew I was lacto-vegetarian for life."

Newsletters and magazines can also be effective in changing people's behaviour. For example, on issue of the "People for the Ethical Treatment of Animals News' had an immediate and powerful impact on several people we spoke with. George described his reaction, "I stopped eating meat and fish exactly one year ago, on the day I received volume one, number eight of the publication, PETA news. One of the articles was titled "Downed Cow". That particular article changed my life. That entire issue was shocking, sad, and the reason I will never eat meat again."

The above quotations indicate that books and other publications are important motivators of change for some people. In addition, many people rely heavily on books and other literature for information and encouragement after become vegetarian. Books containing information on vegetarian nutrition, for example are often sought out, as we discuss later. And new cook-books are a necessity, as most neophytes quickly discover that that their old meat centered cook books are limited. Not only do traditional cook books have few recipes that feature plant foods as main courses, but the vegetable dishes they do include are generally unimaginative and dull. Many people report that exploring new recipes in vegetarian cook books is one of the most enjoyable aspects of this period.

Vegetarian literature is particularly important for those who do not know other vegetarians personally. For these people having a subscription to magazine such as *Vegetarian Times* or a vegetarian newsletter reduces feelings of isolation. A subscription also provides support and helps them to stick with a difficult decision when the going gets rough. Vegetarian not only is a catalyst for behaviour change, but also plays a role in maintaining that change over time.

New Research

Many people argue that, unlike people, non-human animals are incapable of feeling pain. However, evidence from three sources indicates that most animals are as capable of suffering as are humans.

First, research in comparative neuropsychology indicates that there are *no significant structural differences* between the nervous systems of humans and other animals. Instead, the mechanisms of pain perception, including the sensory receptors in the skin, the neural pathways that convey pain messages to the central nervous system, and the brain structures that "register" pain, are common to most species. This reflects our common evolutionary history. It is true that humans, compared with most other animals, have a large cerebral cortex—the part of the brain used for higher thought. But this difference is one of degree rather than kind. As Brian Kolb and Lan Whishaw, two neuropsychologist, point out:

To many people, including many psychologists, both human neuroanatomy and human cognitive processes (i.e., thinking) fundamentally differ from those of animals. After all, humans talk, read, write and do all sorts of things that no monkey or meat has ever done. It is our view that this line of reasoning is shortsighted and wrong. There is no compelling evidence that there is a qualitative difference between the brains of humans and those of other animals.

Second, behavioral studies reveal that animals and humans *react in similar ways* to aversive stimuli such as electric shocks or burns: that is, they cry out and try to escape. Like humans, animals in pain also secrete adrenaline and reveal metabolic activity. However, when animals are given pain-killing drugs they do not exhibit these reactions. Similarly, if injured, both humans and animals will clutch a damaged limb and keep it still. And animals, like humans, learn to avoid behaviors that are physically punished. These common behaviours indicate that nonhuman animals do not like pain any more than humans do.

Third, the theory of evolution holds that the experience of pain has survival value for a species in that it informs individuals that they are in danger (for example, when being attacked) and that they should escape as quickly as possible. Pain also teaches animals about aversive and potentially dangerous things, such as, fire should be avoided. Because the ability to suffer is adaptive, pain is likely to be experienced by all living things with highly developed nervous systems that have some degree of control over their environments and are capable of moving from one place to another. This, of course, would include most animals and fish but would exclude all plants. (Plants have no nervous systems and so cannot experience pain. And because they cannot escape from danger the ability to perceive pain confers no evolutionary advantage) In addition, the fact that many species of plants involve thorns, barbs, and needles as forms of protection is also informative for they would only be effective against animals capable of feeling pain.

Many argue that humans are more intelligent than animals. Although this is certainly true, recent research reveals that animals are more intelligent than previously believed. Animals of many species are capable of making and using tools, have elaborate communication systems, live in completely organized societies, cooperate to achieve common goals, and help one another. Furthermore, much of the behaviour of animals is learned-not guided by instinct as was once thought. Most animals are capable of learning new skills and can even teach these to their offspring. Many people, for example, would be aware of recent studies in which rudimentary American sign language has been successfully taught to a variety of primates, including chimpanzees, gorillas, and orangutans. Chimpanzee mothers have been observed teaching many of these signs to their children.

Some people argue that animals are incapable of making free choices. But animals do appear to show preferences for things and to act on the basis of plans and goals. Research on problem-solving in higher mammals, such as chimpanzees, indicates that they are capable of planning and carrying out complete sequence of activities to achieve a reward, such as food. Indeed, one might ask, who is more goal-directed—the lioness who stocks her meat or the man who treads the well-beaten path from the television to the refrigerator for his next beer?

Few people subscribe to the morality that inaction is permissible simply because one possesses the power to carry it out. As Mohandas Gandhi argued the fact that we are more intelligent than animals and have power over them does not give us the right to exploit them. To the contrary, we are obligated to protect them. For individuals who agree with these ethical arguments, vegetarianism is mandatory.

Darwin's View

Modern ethical vegetarianism also owes a debate to Charles Darwin, who like Jeremy Bentham, provided philosophical weight to the conviction that animals deserve, our respect whilst failing to take personal note of his own conclusions. Darwin's theory of evolution emphasized that, there is no fundamental difference between man and the higher mammals. Dombrowski summarizes the implications of this as follows:

> Animals feel pain, love, have the desire to be loved, suffer from ennui, have dreams, and for all we know, may be self conscious as well as conscious. Although animals do not have the ennobling belief in God, many human beings do not have this belief either (nor do some men have reasons, and we do not (or should not) kill and eat them... Once the weight of evidence in favour of Darwin's theory become apparent, practically every earlier justification of man's supreme place in creating and his dominion over the animals had to be rejected. Darwin signals a revolution in our perception of animals: we are animals!

It was said by Henry Salt, an Eton housemaster who was one of the first modern champions of vegetarianism in his pamphlet the logic of Vegetarianism that success in what he termed 'the reform of diet' depended on a sincere belief in the moral rightness of the cause. His point was that all the arguments in favour of vegetarianism in the end reflect a fundamental ethical position and it is this that gives the logic of vegetarianism its force. '*The spirit* in which one takes up vegetarianism', Salt concluded, 'is the main factor in the result. It is useless to look for any absolute proof in such matters—the proof is in one's self—for those, at least, who have heart to feel, and brain to ponder the cruelty and folly of flesh-eating.

Religious Reasons

As already discussed, religious beliefs, or a desire to live a more spiritual life, constitute another important motive for abstaining from flesh. Religious vegetarian can be divided into three groups. First, some people belong to religious groups in which vegetarianism is either required (such as the

International Society for Krishna Consciousness) or strongly recommended (such as the Seventh-Day Adventists). In most cases these people give up flesh when they convert to their new faith. Second, some people belong to religions that do not have a strong vegetarian tradition, such as Catholicism or Judaism. Nevertheless, these people feel that a meatless diet is consistent with the ethical teachings of their religions. Third, some people do not belong to a formal organized religion, but believe that a meatless diet allows them to live a more spiritual existence.

Many Eastern religions, discourage the eating of meat because it is believed that animals, as well as humans, have souls. Because of this killing and eating animals incurs a moral debt that a person must one day repay. We spoke with several members of the International Society for Krishna Consciousness who explained their personal reasons for being vegetarians. Some worried about the negative consequences of eating animals. Whereas others felt that a vegetarian diet makes one more receptive to spiritual values. One such person opines, "When I joined the Hare Krishna movement I learned about the violent slaughter of animals and the Karmic effects of eating meat. The reason for the diet is to lessen the *karma*, so you can get out of this cycle of death and rebirth. I became a Hare Krishna devotee and, of course, the Vedic scriptures are insistent about being a vegetarian. Giving up the eating of meat helps clear the mind and open the heart to religious ideas.

Followers of Sri Chinmoy—a religious teacher from India, are also vegetarian. Sujantra, a member of the Sri Chinmoy group explained his reasons for not eating meat; "I've found that the vibrations of food affect my nerves on a very subtle level. It aids your meditation to eat foods that have a milder vibration, like fruits and vegetables and to stay away from foods like meat. In order to meditate and to pray, you don't have to be vegetarian and because someone is a vegetarian doesn't mean that they are any more spiritual than anyone else. Yet, being a vegetarian can enhance your meditation because of the peaceful vibration in the food."

Western religions are also represented among the ranks of religious vegetarians. Several people in our sample were Seventh-Day Adventists—a religious group with a strong vegetarian tradition. Seventh-Day Adventists believe that meat, particularly meat produced by factory farm methods, is often tainted with disease and is generally unhealthy. Because Christians should maintain good health in order to do Gods work, eating meat is frowned upon by the Church. Tom, a pastor in the Seventh-Day Adventist Church, explained his views on eating flesh. As he pointed out good reasons can be found in the Bible to justify a vegetarian diet, "Seventh-Day Adventists get their perspective from the Bible. In the beginning, when God created people, he created them vegetarian. There would be no death, and consequently, there would be no death of animals, so there would be no meat. If you read genealogies up to the flood, you will find that people lived to be seven, eight, nine hundred years old. Right after the flood, you will find that when man was permitted to eat meat, his life expectancy decreased rapidly to three score and ten. It almost looks as if there was a direct relationship between the two. We recognize that there are hundreds of diseases that an animal can have, and many of those can be communicated to humans.... The devil has a three-pronged attack. He's got a poor technology, which will destroy your spiritual life. He also has things that will destroy your mind. And then he has things that will destroy your body. Meat is one of them. So we encourage people to be vegetarian."

Mormons are not allowed to drink alcohol or to smoke. Steve, a Mormon, believed that his religion also required him to be a vegetarian. He explains, "I first gave up meat because our religion asks us to eat meat only if we need to sustain ourselves. In the doctrines and covenants which the Mormons would consider to be a revelation from Jesus Christ through

Joseph Smith-it says that if is pleasing to the Lord to eat meat only in times of cold winter of famine. I interpret that to mean that we should eat meat only to sustain ourselves when we can't get other food."

However, Steve admitted that few people in his church agree with his interpretation of this particular passage. Although many Mormons eat meat in moderation relatively few are true vegetarians.

Some Christians do not belong to church or sect that formally encourages vegetarianism. Nevertheless, many find a meatless diet to be consistent with their own understanding of the Bible and Christ's teachings. Some believe that the treatment of animals in modern factory farms contradicts the Christian values of kindness and compassion. Others feel that killing and eating animals is a violation of the general injunction not to kill unnecessarily. A personal comment of a Christian, "God declared, straight from the Bible, any pork consumption is a sin. He also informed us as to what He allowed us to eat. God intended animal consumption, but never any suffering to any life that He created. Man has decided to make a mockery of God's Commandments. The end result: the hideous suffering of innocent, helpless, beautiful creatures.

l always quote the ten commandments. Thou shalt not kill. It doesn't say kill what. It just says thou shalt not kill. But these people who enjoy meat change the ruler around to say that God didn't mean animals—only people."

Finally, as noted above, some religious vegetarians do not belong to any particular religion—East or West-or adhere to any particular doctrine. Nevertheless, they feel that being vegetarian allows them to achieve a more spiritual life than would otherwise be possible. To some, the killing of animals for food—an act of violence—is incompatible with higher spiritual ideals. Others believe that eating meat stimulates base, carnal desires.

Beliefs of religious vegetarians are diverse, with some drawing their inspiration primarily from Eastern religions and others adhering more to Western religions. But in spite of their diversity of views, they all share a belief the being a vegetarian is good for the soul and brings one closer to God.

Ecological and Economical Reason

For a few people, the initial reasons for giving up meat have less to do with their beliefs and values and more to do with harsh economic realities. Meat is a relatively expensive food item. Because of this, some people have their first encounter with vegetarianism during a period of poverty when they cannot afford to buy meat.

Turning to vegetarianism people soon discover other benefits of a meatless diet and continue to live as vegetarians after their financial situations improve.

Animals are economically and ecologically expensive food sources and the continuing emphasis on meat as a staple commodity is in fact a contributory factor in world hunger. Cattle, in the words of Frances Moore Lappe, are 'protein factories in reverse'. She points out that it takes approximately units of plant protein to yields 1 unit of animal protein: the remaining 7 units are needed by the animal for its own biological processes.

Ecology/Environment

Some people come to vegetarianism via the environmental movement. These "environmental vegetarians" are sometimes conservationists directly involved in preserving our wildlife. Some are members of Green Peace or other activist environmental groups. For these people, the main reason for adopting a vegetarian diet is to minimize the destructive effects of livestock production on our soil, water, forests, and wildlife. As a commercial artist, wrote; "My concern for the environment is what keeps me going. I'm saying "No" to the fast food hamburger chains, destruction of rainforest for grazing land, "No" to overgrazing the continent of Africa and the resulting starvation of millions, and "No" to the human aggression toward all living creatures."

- Two hundred years ago, American cropland had topsoil that averaged 21 inches in depth. Today, only about 6 inches remain. Every year in the US an area the size of Connecticut is lost to topsoil erosion—85% of this erosion is associated with livestock production.

Put another way, livestock animals on average consume 20 pounds of plant protein for every pound of meat they yield; which clearly shows that it is plant proteins not animal that have the real potential for alleviating the worlds food problems. A plant creates its protein from water, carbon dioxide and nitrogen: animals have to eat plants or other animals to get their protein. A cow can certainly convert plant foods into protein for human consumption, but at huge cost, both in financial and human terms. These are not new ideas: they have long been recognized and the gross inefficiency of meat production articulated many times over the last decade or so. The link between agricultural inefficiency and global food shortages was pointed out by Senator Hubert Humphrey in 1974, in a speech at the Remselaer Conference on world Hunger at the United Nations: 'A decision by Americans to eat one less hamburger each week would make some 10 million tons of grain available for food assistance to the world'. A year later, in 1975, the English author Jon Wyme Tyson wrote: 'We read in our newspapers about the starving and under-fed millions, and all the time we are feeding to meat producing animals the very crops the could more than eradicate world food shortage: also, we are importing from starving nations large quantities of grain and other foods that are then fed to our animals instead of to the populations who produced them.

But little has changed. Well over 350 million tons of the world's grain harvest is fed to animals every year while some 350 million of the world's children are suffering from malnutrition. Meat is still reared and consumed in vast quantities; the hopeless million still starve.

- Every six seconds someone in the world starves to death, that is, between 10,000 and 14,000 people a day or three and a half million a year. The American experience again points up the iniquities of a national diet based on meat. In America, each person is fed by 5 acres of land and the average American consumes 300 pounds of meat per year. This means the some 45 per cent of American arable land is given over to graze livestock, whilst only 17 per cent is used for crops: 'During the final four months of a steer's life, through overfeeding he gains 600 to 800 pounds. During this time he consumes over a ton of feed. Multiply that by the millions of steers all munching away at once, and you've got a situation in which livestock consume 97 per cent of the nation's legumes, 90 per cent of its grain and 80 per cent of its fish.

There are other undesirable spin-offs from meat production on a large scale besides the scandalous squandering of land and crop resources. The intensive rearing of animal for meat requires immense amounts of water for the irrigation of crops to feed livestock, drinking water for the animals and the water used in meat production. In total, to sustain a meat diet requires eight times more water than it would to support a plant-based diet.

- At the same time that meat production *uses* water on a massive scale, also *polluting* it. The waste matter produced by slaughterhouses—fat, grease, offal, faecal matter, carcases etc.—can create local pollution: but the main problem concerns livestock waste, which is a widespread cause of water pollution. (One might think that it would be logical to use such waste as fertilizer: but in practice it is often cheaper to use chemical fertilizers.) For example, in America many of the areas with water pollution problems are located near areas of intensive livestock rearing (Oklahoma, Kansas, Illinois, the Ohio Valley, the Texas Panhandle).

- Deforestation is another problem associated with a high demand for meat because of the conversion of forest to grazing land for livestock. In Latin America one of the prime factors in the terrible acceleration of deforestation is the demand for grazing land for cattle. Between 1950 and 1975 the area of man-established pasture in Central America more than doubled mostly as a result of clearing tropical forests: 'The major causes of deforestation in the world are inextricably linked to the production of animal foods' especially meat and the grazing land experience a crisis in the need for forest products in another generation on two.

- Soil erosion is yet another concomitant of an agricultural economy based on livestock. Throughout history, overgrazing has had serious environmental consequences: this is still a problem, even in developed countries. According to John Block, President Reagan's Secretary of Agriculture, the USA is facing a soil erosion crisis with 60 per cent of its rangelands being overgrazed. Million of acres of land are lost each year both in America and elsewhere, as a result of soil erosion, much of which is attributable to livestock agriculture. It has been calculated that a vegetarian economy would eliminate as much as 90 per cent of this erosion.

Cattle are inefficient food sources on a small scale as well as a large scale:

> "It takes maybe 1½ acres of land to feed an adult on grains and vegetables, but you'll probably have to set aside about 20 acres to feed and graze a cow. Even the cost of refrigeration is something we don't want to contend with. As far as I'm concerned their biggest use lies in their ability to replace a tractor and to give manure and milk. The meat industry is built on tipsy-turvy economic principles. Massive wastage is taken for granted. One estimate puts losses due to disease in British pigs at 137 million pounds a year, 33 million to 'unplanned deaths', 94 million to 'lost production potential', and 10 million to vet and drugs bills. These losses average nearly 10 per pig."

Or take beef cattle, 1200lb of protein a year is required to produce 75lb of meat protein and this is for an intensively reared beast:

A grazing steer will produce only 5lb of protein per acre of land and is hopelessly inefficient unless the land is unsuited to any other use. If however you put the steers in a bean and feed them on barley grown on that same acre of land you can produce 50lb of protein. Grow wheat instead and forget about the steer altogether and you get 185lb of protein from your acre of land. Switch to growing soy and you could increase the acreage yield to 560lb of protein, ten times that best yield that factory farming can produce."

Factory Farming

Meat in the latter half of the twentieth century is far removed from the tabled 'roast beef of old England'. By the time it reaches the table it has been through a bewildering variety of processes to make it conform to marketing requirements which spuriously reflect 'what the customer wants'. The long-term effects of such processes are unknown; but already the signs are that they are having undesirable consequences.

The idea of animals being reared for the table in gentle pastoral surroundings is a myth as far as the modern meat industry is concerned. Animal welfare and the profit motive are incompatible. Impersonal, not to say ruthless, corporate logic requires a systematized production line. There is no room for sentimentality, or even simple compassion, down on the factory farm. Let's pause for a moment and remind ourselves what the intensive rearing of animals involves.

- Even today, with the proliferation of free range eggs, most of our eggs come from hens that spend miserable lives imprisoned in cages that allow them no room to move. Their natural behaviour patterns are completely destroyed and after about fifteen months they are thrown out to be slaughtered, often featherless blind and lame from their imprisonment. The battery system produces birds that are never allowed to run, scratch the ground, or make a dust bath as they would in a natural environment. They never spread their wings; they never relate to other members of their own species; they can never fulfill their internal instincts which are highly developed in hens. The average wing span of a chicken is 32 inches, but they are generally allowed only 4 inches of cage width per bird in battery houses. In order to stimulate egg production the light intensity in a battery house is maintained for anything up to 18 hours a day. Because of boredom, pecking and even cannibalism is common which leads to de-beaking of the birds. Hens kept in these conditions produce eggs that often differ in nutritional quality from free range eggs.

- It is not unusual in today's factory henhouse for 4 or 5 hens to be squeezed into a 12" x 18" cage. It is standard for poultry producers to de-beak chicks with hot-knife machines—not a painless procedure. De-beaking is industry's solution to birds, driven to crazed pecking, inflicting harm upon the fellow "product."

Once again wastage is an accepted fact of life. It is not unusual for battery egg operation to lose between 10 and 15 per cent of its hens a year, mostly from problems related to the overcrowded and unnatural conditions: 'According to the manager of a 50,000 bird egg ranch [in Madhya Pradesh] five to ten of his hens succumb daily to confinement stress. (That's between two to four thousand per year.) "Those birds," he says, "don't die of any disease. They just can't take the stress of crowded living."

- In egg factories all over the country, male chicks are weeded out and disposed of by "chick-pullers." Over half a million chicks a day are stuffed en masse into plastic bags where they are crushed and suffocated. Or they may be ground up while still alive to be fed to livestock or used as fertilizer.

Peter Singer has pointed out that 'of all the animals commonly eaten in the Western world' the pig is without doubt the most intelligent. When George Orwell put the pigs in charge of Animal Farm his choice was defensible on scientific as well as literary grounds'. As a consequence of its intelligence a pig is particularly sensitive to its environment and social setting. When they are intensively reared boredom is a very real problem. In confined conditions pigs start to bite each other's tails (the common remedy for which is tail-docking) and they suffer from acute stress, as mentioned earlier (see p.34). Sows spend their pregnancies in what are called dry-sow stalls. They are forced to lie on concrete floors, slatted at the rear to allow dung and urine to fall through. The slats cause soreness to the back feet of the sow. Because of the construction of the stalls lameness and spinal troubles are common. When they are ready to farrow the sows are moved to farrowing pens, which are similarly constructed. Seven days after farrowing the litters are taken away from the sows, who will be stocked again and put back into the dry row stalls. As for the piglets, when they are two to three weeks old they are put into battery cages, three tiers high, where they remain until they reach about 100lb live weight. They are then fattened in pens.

Back in 1965 the Brambell Report recommended a mandatory safeguard for pigs: 'Pregnant sows should not be kept without daily exercise in quarters which do not permit them to turn around and, in any case, should not be tethered indoors.' The practice of intensive close confining of pigs still goes on. One little regarded aspect of the intensive process is the consequences of fire on factory farms. Statistics are hard to come by, but in 1979 compassion in World Farming quoted a Fire Research Memorandum that estimated that in a single year 200,000 head of livestock were burnt to death while trapped in their cages or stalls.

The same organization provided the following summary of factory farm animals. They compete directly with man for food consuming oilseed proteins needed in countries where they are grown in the fight against malnutrition; create the need for continuous corn growing, which in turn calls for more chemical fertilizers, weed-killers and pesticides to the detriment of the wildlife of the countryside;

- waste primary food (only 10 per-cent efficiency);
- cause air and water pollution;
- degrade the sensibilities of all who work with them and threaten health because of the drug residues and pathogens which they pass on in their products and meat.

The 1965 Brambell Report, mentioned earlier, is a seminal document in the modern literature of animal welfare and is still of great interest to all vegetarians. The committee was set up under F.W. Rogers Brambell, a distinguished zoologist, and included an appendix by W.H. Thorpe, Director of the Department of Animal Behaviour at Cambridge (It is interesting to note that the first Professorship of Animal Welfare is being established at Cambridge, as a result of a recognition of the need to promote studies into animal health, the ethical considerations arising from the role of animals in society and the codes of practice in animal production. In 1985 the clinical veterinary Medicine Syndicate at Cambridge stresses the need for further research into the behavioral and physiological bases of animal stress, aggression and fear research that relates directly to the exploitative methods of intensive farming.) The Brambell Report remains essential reading for anyone interested in animal rights and the barbarities of factory farming. In his appendix Thorpe stresses the effects of intensive reading on animals either used to or conditioned to respond to the freedom of movement and social integration of their natural environments:

"All the domestic animals which man farms are species which, in the wild, show a fairly highly organized social life either in flock, family, clan or herd. This means that behavioural organization is also potentially on a higher level than the ordinary man imagines. Even though a cow in a stall or a pig in a sty may appear stupid enough, this impression may be quite erroneous simply because we have never even begun to comprehend the social organization of the wild ancestor which in turn, despite the effects of domestications, still undoubtedly determines the sensory abilities and level of feeling and perception of the animal.

Chemicals in Meat

In the pursuit of profit, the meat industry relies heavily on chemical additives of various kinds to 'improve' its products for preservation, colouring, texturing, promoting growth, tranquillizing and keeping unprofitable illnesses at bay.

Cattle do not roam soft rolling hillsides, contentedly chewing the cud before being humanely dispatched, as some meat-eaters still fondly believe, or try to believe. From birth they are given antibiotics, tranquillizers, and hormones: after slaughtering their carcasses are injected with more chemical agents: colouring agents to make decomposing flesh look 'appetizing' and 'fresh'; sodium nitrite and sodium nitrate to arrest the rate of putrefaction (Under certain conditions, nitrites combine with amines found in meats and other foods, such as wine and beer, to form nitrosamines called by the F.D.A. [Food and Drugs Administration] "One of the most formidable and versatile groups of carcinogens yet discovered).

The greatest hygiene risks occur during slaughter and dressing and result not only from disease but also from the techniques used, the spillage of contaminated matter, contact with the outer hide or skin of the slaughtered animals, regurgitated stomach contents and fecal matter. Particular causes for concern include inadequately cleaned sticking Knives and pitching rods, incorrect flaying, soiling of the carcasses and problems with the skimming and 'tailing out' of animals dressed on the floors of slaughter houses.

Few people, even committed vegetarians would care to spend time in an abattoir; but one who has is Dr Alan Long:

The gangs have always invited me to join in their tea-breaks, although I have never been offered clean overalls for my visits (the best advice I received: 'Bring old clothes there's a lot of blood in there'). Hygiene is execrable. Bouts of idiotic and obscene chanting occur in the din. Many slaughter men are defensive over their tasks ("Well it's legal, isn't it?"). Many declare their revulsion at killing calves and horses and at ritual slaughter ('But its all part of the job, isn't it?'). Piece work rates leave very little time for niceties.

Vets and meat-inspectors harden in their attitudes, [one] managed by tenuous recourse to hygiene regulations to forestall a kill of fully conscious sheep by a slaughter man "equipped with nothing more suitable than a blunt bread-knife"

As a consequence of intensive methods of husbandry the meat producers have had to resort to the widespread use of antibiotics to counteract the disease-risks inherent in their methods. It is almost impossible to slaughter animals without substantial levels of contamination. Dr. A. H. Linton of the Bristol University Medical School estimated that at least 52 per cent of bovine carcasses and 83 per cent of pigs carcasses are contaminated by bacteria of the *E.Coli* type, and there is an increasing spread of resistant bacteria and infection of the urinary tract, enteritis in babies, salmonella infections, any cystitis as a result of drug resistant enteric bacteria. Jon Wyme Tyson reminds us that:

> "Decomposition begins as soon as an animal is slaughtered. Its blood stream just like our own' serves as a debris conveyor for toxic wastes. To give our system the additional job of eliminating another creature's unwanted material together with the toxins of fear that are released into its blood stream prior to slaughter seems to suggest at the very least, a very unaesthetic regard for the joys of nutrition."

Flesh foods are nearly always responsible for food poisoning. In 1975 there were 11,000 *reported* cases of salmonella poisoning in the UK. Three years later in 1978, a report by the British Association for the Advancement of Science noted: 'Undoubtedly the greatest dangers arise from conditions in slaughterhouses. Contaminated meat is perhaps the main cause of the pathogen's spread.' This view received tragic confirmation is 1984 when nineteen old people died of food poisoning at the Stanley Royd Hospital in Yorkshire. There had been salmonella outbreaks at the hospital in 1974 and 1979 and in March 1982 mince had been returned from the words as unacceptable: laboratory experiments showed that there would have been a real danger if this had been eaten. The 1984 salmonella contamination infected more than 400 patients and staff. It was originally thought that cold beef had been responsible for the contamination but the subsequent inquiry was told that, though beef may have been a vehicle it was virtually certain that poultry had been the original source of the infection.

There are also indication that infection by beef tapeworms is increasing in the UK. Tapeworm infection was practically unknown before the Second World War, and even now it arouses little publicity because the worms actually do little physical damage to their human hosts despite their horrific size. In 1978 two scientists, Dr William Crewe and Dr Roderick Owen, both of the Liverpool School of Tropical Medicine, published, an article on beef tapeworms in *New Scientist*. Though the symptoms of beef tapeworm infection in humans are comparatively mild, even with worms that exceed forty feet, the situations is obviously not a desirable one 'The implications are, said the article, 'that a considerable reservoir of tapeworm infection has already established itself in Britain,.

Meat, then, contains two broad categories of contaminant those introduced by meat producers, such as growing boosters (hormones), antibiotics and tranquillizers and naturally occurring pollutants the unavoidable by-products of animal metabolism such as lactic and uric acid, neither of which are beneficial for humans (a high concentration of uric acid predisposes towards kidney stones, gout and arthritis) Adrenaline and other hormones released into animals bodies as a result of the terror induced by the slaughterhouse are also passed on to the human consumers of their dead flesh. The American researcher Orville Schell whose four year investigation resulted in a damning indictment of the meat and poultry industry in the USA, detailed in his book *Modern Meat* reveals that nearly half of all antibiotics manufactured go into animals and there is mounting evidence that resistance to antibiotics is being passed on to humans.

- At least 95% of all toxic chemical residues in the American diet come from meat, fish, dairy products and eggs. This is because such residues are stored in fat. Each step up the food chain serves to amplify the consumption of toxins. Fish, especially, have very long food chains. Avoiding fish to avoid toxic residue may not be a sufficient preventative measure, however, as one third of the world's fish catch is fed to livestock. Due to the excessive use of pesticides, insecticides and petrochemical fertilizers on cropland, the injection of hormones and antibiotics into farm animals, and the abundance of PCBs and mercury in our oceans, there is toxicity in the flesh of all animals people eat. More than ever, it is wise to eat "low on the food chain," with plant food being the lowest and safest.

- The treatment of human disease with antibiotics is showing signs of being hampered by the flagrant overuse of antibiotics fed and injected into the animals people eat. Meat-eaters are exacerbating the trend toward human immunity to medicinal drugs just by eating cow's milk, hamburgers and chicken. This ultimately affects everyone, vegetarians and non-vegetarians alike.

Vegetarianism is also advocated by those concerned with the economic pressure of feeding the world's burgeoning population. From the perspective of land use and the efficiency of agriculture, producing meat is much more expensive than producing vegetable foods. A beef cow must be fed 21 pounds of plant protein in order to produce 1 pound of animal protein for human consumption. Fully one half of all the agricultural land in use in the United States in planted with feed crops, most of which are used to produce meat. Our livestock consumes 10 times the amount of grain we eat ourselves.

This means that a great deal of protein is wasted by feeding it to animals and then eating them, rather than using the plant food directly. Though this same pattern is common in many of the developed countries of the world, The United States is the most extreme example. It has been estimated that with what they waste in their country alone, through meat consumption, 90% of the protein for the entire world could be met. If meat were dropped from the diets of the U.S. and a few other countries, everyone on earth could eat well.

Environmental Toxins and the Vegetarian Diet

Plants are the basis of all human nutrition. Meat is second hand, in a sense; it is as a result of animals consuming plants. Next in this chain are those who eat meat, such as carnivorous mammals or birds of prey. Environmental toxins are progressively concentrated as one moves up the food chain as we have also seen in the above discussion.

This happens because animals eating contaminated plants gradually accumulate the toxic materials contained in the plants. By using animals for food, the carnivores who are next up in this sequence find themselves on a diet that contains higher levels of the toxic substances, and as these carnivores accumulate what is present in their prey, concentrations in their tissues gradually rise, well above those of the animals they eat.

For example, hawks and eagles that live on the flesh of small animals have suffered a reduction in numbers because their eggs would not hatch. This is thought to be due to pesticide residues in the egg. An animal eating a carnivore, being another step further upon the food chain, would be in danger of concentrating even higher levels of poison in its body. It is perhaps for this reason that humans have usually avoided using flesh-eating birds or animals as a source of food. This provides some protection against the intake of toxic,— substances—man-made or naturally occurring that can accumulate in food chains.

A meat-free diet is hence more protective, because eating a predominantly vegetarian diet allows us to eat still lower on the food chain. This is of particular significance if one is concerned about toxic chemicals such as pesticides that may be taken in through the diet.

Pesticides have been used extensively in homes and factories, but because current agricultural practices rely heavily on the use of insecticides and herbicides, their presence in food supplies has been a matter of special concern. Rachel Carson first called attention to the problem in 1962 in her book *Silent Spring*. Yet the use of agricultural pesticides in the United States has increased from 200000 pounds per year in the 1950s to 1.1 billion pounds today. Fortunately according to a recent news report, less than 2% of plant foods tested are above the suggested tolerance levels for residues. Animal foods, on the other hand, reflect their position on the food chain and their tendency to concentrate chemicals from the plants or animals they eat: pesticide levels in them are considerably higher.

Insecticides are of two major classes: chlorinated hydrocarbons, typified by DDT and organophosphates, which have been used as never poisons in chemical warfare and which have been marketed recently under such names as malathion.

DDT and DDT Derivatives as an Example of Pesticide Residues in Common Foods.

DDT, like the other chemicals in its class, is a relatively stable compound, so it persists for quite a long time. After crops are sprayed with it, it will turn up in the soil or food supplies years later. DDT and the other chlorinated hydrocarbon pesticides had been discontinued or severely restricted by the end of the 1970s.

Though they have now been replaced by less persistent chemicals that do not tend to accumulate in the environment, residues of them still turn up. Since they are fat soluble, they are especially high in foods containing animal fats. Yet studies do show that their levels are decreasing, and over a period of years they should slowly disappear from our food supplies. The newer organophosphates such as malathion, shorter lived but perhaps more toxic, have been found in vegetable oils and in oranges and apples, but levels have been well within the limits of what is considered safe. (these pesticide polluted crop is when fed to animals which are in turn consumed by humans leads to bio-concentration of these chemicals leading to many untoward effects.)

More troublesome in a way than the pesticides are the notorious PCBs and PBBs industrial chemicals that have escaped into the environment. They are not biodegradable at all and are therefore even more persistent than DDT, tendig to float about in the air, water, and food supply indefinitely. Moreover, they are toxic at considerably lower doses than DDT.

The United States Food and Drug Administration set a maximum permissible PCB level of five parts per million in fish. But breast milk of mothers living in industrial areas has commonly shown levels this high and higher. Like DDT and other similar compounds, PCBs, accumulate in food chains, so there is concern about their cumulative toxicity. Exposure to high doses has led to an increased rate of liver cancer, but experts feel that at the levels usually present PCBs do not in and of themselves make a major contribution to the incidence of cancer in the population at large. There remains, nevertheless, the possibility that they might act synergistically with other cancer-causing agents and thereby increase risk. PBBs (Polybrominatedbiphenyls) had dramatically into the news as a result of the "Fire master incident" in Michigan in 1973. A truck driver accidentally delivered to a manufacturer of animal feeds 2000 pounds of a fire retardant based on PBBs, instead of the expected magnesium supplement. The fire retardant containing the toxic chemical was added to the feed and distributed to hundreds of farms in Michigan. As a result, thousand of animals died and there have been disturbing levels of PBBs in the Michigan food supplies for some years. Fortunately the Fire master disaster was a local one, and, unlike PCBs, PBBs are not widespread environmental contaminate.

Other environmental toxins of concern that find their way into the food supply are those that are present primarily in meat, such as DES, which will be discussed in the next chapter, and the heavy metals, such as lead and mercury. Mercury is a problem restricted primarily to fish, but lead is much more pervasive, and lead poisoning is thought to be quite common. This is especially true in inner cities, where automobile exhaust fumes from leaded gasoline are concentrated. In American cities, one of every four children is thought to be suffering from lead toxicity. Affecting preferentially the nervous system, lead causes emotional and behavioural problems, and eventually brain damage because of the widespread distribution of lead in the environment that has occurred in modern times. Lead is found at varying levels in the food supply. It accumulates in bone and as a rule is highest in animal foods that may contain some bone fragment such as hamburger. However, shellfish taken from polluted waters have on occasion been found to have extremely high levels. Plant foods generally have little, though wild greens gathered along busy highways may have dangerous levels of lead picked up from automobile exhaust.

Original Motives Change at Times

The original reasons that people have for giving up meat may not be the same reasons they hold for continuing to live as vegetarians. To explore this issue, we asked people if their reasons for being vegetarian had changed in any way since they first stopped eating flesh. As it turns out, most people's reasons do change over time.

The most common pattern is for people to begin with a single motive and later to become aware and accepting of other reasons. Once people stop eating met for whatever motive, curiosity leads them to seek out information on other aspects of vegetarianism. In addition, questions and criticisms from meat-eaters lead many vegetarians to become better informed about the issues involved. As they do this, they discover new reasons for abstaining from meat for many, these new reasons become more compelling than the original ones.

Some people start off for reasons of health or other personal benefits and later come to appreciate the ethical and social implications of what they are doing. Note the comments of one person, "I originally gave up animal foods for health and nutritional reasons. But the longer I remain vegan, the more I'm seeing that the eating of animal and animal by-products is morally wrong as well.

I became vegetarian as a New Year's resolution. Three months later I attended an animal rights meeting and I walked out a vegan. My previous health reasons for abstaining from animal flesh quickly turned into a total, new ethical consideration of my diet and lifestyle."

It means early experimentation with a meatless diet can later grow into a deep and personal commitment. This level of commitment is often unanticipated by the no vice vegetarian.

Some other cases, people who originally become vegetarian out of a concern for animals or other social issues discover that personal health benefits are also important reasons for continuing a fleshless diet. One such vegetarian admits.

> "My first reason was simply compassion for animals. But since my original revelations my reasons have expanded and grown. Most meat is full of hormones, pesticide residues, large amounts of fat and little dietary fiber so health reasons have also come into play. I became a lacto-vegetarian strictly for moral and ethical reasons. I truthfully was unaware of the health problems involved in meat-eating until long after I had launched into vegetarianism. I had given no thought to the chemicals applied to animals which soak thought to their skin or the chemicals added to their feed to make them fat. Now I wonder how anyone can eat meat regardless of now they feel about animals. To me meat is the unhealthiest food that can go into the body."

When people adopt new reasons, they are more likely to change from a concern with personal benefits to a concern with ethical social issues as they are to do the reverse. This suggests a natural progression for people who originally stop eating meat for their own self-interest later to come to appreciate the larger ethical and social implications of their actions. In contrast, those who originally become vegetarian for altruistic reasons are less likely to explore, or acknowledge, the beneficial effects for themselves. Perhaps this is because people with strong ethical motives tend to be less concerned with personal gain than others are. Alternatively, it may be that ethical vegetarians feel that explicitly accepting the personal benefits of a meatless diet might compromise the integrity and purity of their stand.

Another common pattern is for people not to change their initial reasons, but to become more certain of their beliefs and stronger in their convictions over time.

A few long-term vegetarians become so certain of their beliefs, and so committed to their lifestyles, that they rarely think about it any more. It appears that the motives of these people are taken of 15 years, said.

Time for Change

The time taken to make the transition from being a meat-eater to a vegetarian varies considerably. Some stop immediately on the day they decide to become vegetarians while others eliminate meat from their diets over periods of months or even years. A gradual phasing out of meat is the most common approach, with 70 per cent of people taking this route and 30 per cent giving up meat all at once.

Although initial cravings for meant are common, they typically fade with the passing of time—usually within six months to a year. As noted above only a handful of the vegetarians were recent converts. After a period of time, even former meat lovers come to find the sight, and particularly the smell of meat to be nauseating. The following comments are from people who experienced strong craving during the early days of their transition, "vegetarianism gets easier all the time the farther away I get from flesh eating, the more repulsive it seems."

Now the smell of hamburger cooking alone upsets my stomach, and I do not like going into restaurants. The business of dining strikes me as some what decadent especially when the dined-upon are dead animals"

"In this stage of my conservation, I can't stand the smell of any flesh food and become nauseated at the thought of eating it."

To further explore this issue, we asked people how they would feel about eating meat now. This turned out to be one of the few questions on which a clear majority emerged: Eighty two per cent of vegetarians say there is no way they would consider eating flesh again. Feelings of disgust at the very thought of eating meat are prominent in most people's response. To many, the idea is simply unthinkable.

Some people are particularly advent about never eating meat again. For example, one person said, "You couldn't get me to eat meat with a gun to my head." Another said, "Someone could pay me a million dollars and I wouldn't do it." Typically, these people have been vegetarian for a relatively long period of time. To them, eating meat has become an impossibility.

Some people no longer think of meat as food. For example, one person said that his eating meat would be equivalent to a meat-eater eating wood; it simply is not an edible thing as far as he concerned. Along similar lines others feel that eating meat is a form of cannibalism; consequently, they do not think about eating animal flesh many more than the average person contemplates eating another human being. For example, Mary, a social worker, said, "If you offered me meat, I'd feel the same as if you barbecued my next door neighbour and offered me a piece of his flesh-totally repulsedy. For those ethical and spiritual vegetarians who feel a deep bond with animals the use of the term "cannibalism" is more than a metaphor—It reflects a belief that the eating of animal flesh and the eating of human flesh are equally barbaric.

In spite of the fact that most vegetarians feel so strongly about never eating meat again, a minority (17%) say they might under certain circumstance. For example, a few claim they will politely eat meat if it is served to them by relatives. And a few recent converts admit that they wouldn't mind trying some of their favorite meat dishes gain. Jamie, a raw foodist said that people shouldn't make a "religion" out of vegetarianism and that he would have no qualms about eating meat again, if he had the urge. However, he pointed out that if he were to eat meat, it would have to be raw!

In summary, for most people, the transition to vegetarianism is a major life change. Initially, the novelty can be overwhelming. Many new vegetarians are not 100 per cent confident that they have made the right decision and have doubts about their will power. Some anticipate symptoms of meat withdrawal or near starvation because they do not know what to cook. Others worry that they will become weak and anemic. And most feel awkward calling themselves "vegetarians' when only a short time ago they were gnawing on drumsticks, Giving up flesh involves more than simply buying a new cook book; it involves a major shift in one's self-concept and life-style. As part of this process, new vegetarians have to relearn many of their beliefs, attitudes, and behaviour.

However, at the same time, there is a sense of adventure and fun, in becoming a vegetarian. And typically, over the course of a year or so, people adapt. They learn how to cook, establish new eating habits, and lose their anxiety about whether or not they made the right choice. At a certain point, the inevitable happens: people become "real" vegetarians. After this, it feels normal to abstain from flesh, and without any self consciousness, people define them-selves as vegetarians. When someone looks at a steak and thinks, "My God, How can people eat that staff?" It is clear that the transition has been successful.

Instantaneous Change

Individuals who give up meat suddenly fall into four categories. First, those who have experiences that evoke strong emotional reactions change quickly. Meat insight experiences, for example, can produce feelings of disgust that lead people to become vegetarians on the spot. Others feel such moral outrage after learning about conditions on factory farms that they now without further consideration never to eat meat again. Mike, a high school teacher, told us that he had never considered vegetarianism before receiving an issue of PETA News dealing with farm animals.

I quit on the spot, totally. Before I received that issue (out of the blue I might add—I must have been on a mailing list), I had eaten a cheeseburger for lunch. When I got up from my reading chair I was a vegetarian and haven't eaten another creature's body since.

Second, some people what to become vegetarian for a period of time but confront practical barriers that make it difficult for them to stop eating meat. In these cases, people turn vegetarian as soon as their circumstances change. Typical situations are one's in which young adults are living with meat-eating parents or in dormitories. In other cases, people become vegetarians after separating form meat-eating spouses.

Third, some individual plan on becoming vegetarians for a period of time, but wait for a day that implies a clear demarcation between one period and the next to begin. Some people begin their vegetarian diets as a New Year's Eve resolution. Two of our respondents chose Meat Boycott Week to make the change. And moving was good cutting point for Rehman.

The decision to make a commitment to vegetarianism as part of a more general commitment to animals came upon me suddenly. I was moving from one apartment to another, and my brother was helping me. Since our kitchen things were packed up, he went out and got some fast-food fried chicken. I ate the greasy stuff and then announced, "That's it. No more". The repugnance I felt was both physical and moral.

Fourth a few people think about vegetarianism for a long time, but do little about it. Then on a day when they finally feel ready, they announce to the world and to themselves, that they are vegetarians. For these people, the time simply has to be right. As Ashok put it, "Since childhood, I was always bothered by the thought of eating animals. One day, out of nowhere, I decided that I had a choice. I stopped completely"

The Change over Period of Time

As noted earlier, most people make the transition to vegetarianism by gradually eliminating flesh foods from their diets. These periods of time range, in our sample, from one month to four years, with one year being the median amount of time taken. There is a typical pattern to this transition with 79 per cent giving up red meat first, followed by chicken and fish at a later point in time. Some of these people give up red meat and chicken quickly, but continue to eat fish for a relatively longer period of time. Another 12 per cent gradually cut down on all types of meat simultaneously. (In addition, one person who developed an aversion to meat while gnawing on chicken legs gave up those first, one person concerned about the clubbing of baby seals gave up fish first, and one person gave up seal first.)

Quite a few people are eating less meat these days than they did in the past consequently; some individuals notice that their diets have been gradually evolving in the direction of vegetarianism for a long period of time. When these people finally decide to become full vegetarians, the transition is relatively easy because they are already halfway toward their goal. The experience of Jyoti Kaur, mother of two children, "I wanted to get my family off the ground beef merry go round" for health reasons. I had stopped cooking beef and I never bought pork. I made recipes using small portions of chicken and other low fat products. I was trying to get the fat out of our diet. Looking back I realize that I was heading in the direction of vegetarianism, all along. I had taken several steps already, so the final one to a non-flesh lifestyle was easy.

One might predict that people with a strong ethical basis for their beliefs would be more likely to make a quick transition than would those who reject meat for reasons of health or personal growth. However there doesn't appear to be any relation between people's motives for being vegetarian and the length of time it takes them to change. Ethical vegetarians, in fact, often take a relatively long period of time to completely purge flesh from their diets. It seems surprising that the following person took so long to change, considering the strength of her convictions. But her story is not a typical.

For the past two years, I had been heavily involved in the Animal Rights Movement. But it took me a full two years before I stopped eating dead animals. I wonder sometimes why it took me a while, particularly since I knew the truth about where the flesh came from.

Thus, through the experience of all these persons we get a fair idea about what causes conversion to vegetarianism and how permanent the change is.

5

Health Benefits of Vegetarianism and Health Hazards of a Non-Vegetarian Diet

We have seen that why people opt for a vegetarian diet in the preceding discussion. Here we would like to give across the health benefits of a vegetarian diet and qualities of food of plant origin.

Meat contains high proportion of its calories in the form of fat. Though meat is a rich source of energy, people consuming meat regularly get more of it than they need. Excessive quantity of a nutrient needed by the body is harmful for the body. Meat also has a good deal of cholesterol in it. But the much needed fiber context is missing from it. This makes meat a dangerous disease oriented food. Some diseases that are more pronounced in the flesh-eating population and less so in vegetarian societies are discussed below.

Diseases and Diet

Heart Diseases

There are various risk factors for heart diseases. These include life style (sedentary habits, alcohol consumption, high fat and carbohydrate diet, obesity, familial reasons and others)

An impressive example of the benefits of a vegetarian diet is its effect on coronary heart disease. Any measure that can help to prevent this disease deserves attention, since heart diseases are becoming major health problem in India today.

Vegetarians have lower levels of certain risk factors for heart disease such as total serum cholesterol, triglycerides, and low density lipo-proteins. An improvement in risk factors should mean less heart disease. As early as 1961 one physician was bold enough to write in the *Journal of the American Medical Association* that "97% of coronary occlusions (resulting in heart attacks) could be prevented by a vegetarian diet." At that time there was little evidence to back up such a statement, best over the years a number of research papers have been published that put this claim on an increasingly solid foundation in fact. Some of them have looked at directly at heart disease in vegetarians and found it to be decreased, while others provide supporting data.

One recently completed study of 25,000 Californians carried out over a 20-year period showed that meat consumption was associated with a higher incidence of total heart attacks in both men and women. Elaborate statistical analyses indicated that these effects were not due to differences in tobacco use, obesity, or the consumption of other foods besides meat and poultry. The results suggest close-response relationship between meat consumption and heart disease; the more meat eaten, the more heart disease. The difference was most pronounced in men of middle age. For men 45 to 64, there were more than three times as many fatal heart attacks in those who ate meat and poultry than there were in those who were vegetarian.

Countries like New Zealand, Australia, United States and Finland are countries with the highest consumption of animal fats. These are also the countries with the highest rate of mortality from heart disease. The coronary heart disease is in fact the leading killer in the USA. It accounts for close to a million deaths every year.

It is not difficult to locate the reason behind it. Cholesterol present in meat, poultry, seafood, dairy products and eggs leads to build up of plaque in the arteries, causing a atherosclerosis. Saturated fats further increase the alcohol levels. Saturated fats are mainly animal oriented though also present in a few plant-based foods. This build up of plaque in arteries is likely to cause coronary heart disease if the consumption of fatty and cholesterol containing meat is not restricted. American Health Association (AHA) recommends cutting out meat and shifting to plant foods like lentils, beans, tofu etc., in its dietary guidelines. Their study reflects that Vegetarians have lower rates of this fatal heart disease in comparison to meat-eaters. It is on account of lower consumption of cholesterol and fats that vegetarians enjoy better health as compared to meat-eaters. They also have lower blood pressure and lower weight—two more factors that reduce the risk of heart disease.

The beneficial effects on the health of the heart alone should be enough to motivate many people to embark on the transition to vegetarianism. Of course, one should not conclude that heart disease is due solely to diet, or that dietary change alone can prevent it totally. Many other factors have been conclusively shown to contribute to its development, foremost among them cigarette smoking, lack of proper exercise, high blood pressure and hereditary factors.

Hypertension

But it now seems likely that diet can also play a role in the prevention or improvement of high blood pressure. This conclusion emerges from a variety of studies that have looked at the relationship between vegetarianism and blood pressure from a number of different angles. For example, vegetarians have repeatedly been found to have lower blood pressures than those who eat meat, though this difference is probably less dramatic for those who use milk and eggs, and adding meat to the diets of vegetarians raises their blood pressure (hypertension) much less often than meat-eaters; only 2% of vegetarians, compared with 26% of non-vegetarian in one study. Moreover, putting meat-eaters who are hypertensive on a vegetarian diet—even when the diet contains milk and eggs, and salt intake is not reduced—still results in a small but significant decrease in blood pressure. And finally, diets that are essentially vegetarian have been the basis of a number of treatment programmes designed to treat hypertension or reverse coronary heart disease.

Inspite of a favored vegetarian diet I would like to mention here that even an unbalanced vegetarian diet that is rich in saturated fats and has imbalanced nutritional content along with the unhygienic lifestyle can end up in predisposing to the above mentioned disease. hence balanced vegetarian diet helps though not all in all in reduction of the toxic load of the body making it healthier.

(To assess whether a low-fat diet that emphasizes plant-based foods (fruits, vegetables, whole grains, and legumes) was better at lowering cholesterol than a typical low-fat diet, researchers randomly assigned 120 generally healthy adults (age 30–65; 50% men; LDL levels, 130–190 mg/dL; BMI, 19–31) to eat one of these types of diets for 4 weeks.

The two diets were designed to be identical in total fat, saturated fat, protein, carbohydrate, and cholesterol content; and to allow for calorie-intake adjustments to keep body weight constant. Meals either were eaten at the study center or were distributed in coolers to be eaten off site. Fasting blood samples were taken on 4 separate days: 2 at baseline and 2 at study completion.

As expected, body-weight changes were negligible in both groups during the 4-week study. However, compared with the typical low-fat diet, the plant-based low-fat diet yielded significantly greater declines in mean levels of total cholesterol (-17.6 mg/dL vs. -9.2 mg/dL) and of LDL cholesterol (-13.8 mg/dL vs. -7.0 mg/dL). Changes in levels of HDL cholesterol and triglycerides did not differ significantly between the two groups. LDL changes varied widely among individuals.)

Cancer

Both in terms of its direct effects on heart disease and the in-direct benefits that follow reduction in blood pressure, the vegetarian diets seems to hold great promise as a major weapon in the battle against morbidity as well as mortality from cardiovascular disease. Not far behind heart disease, and gaining ground, is cancer. Cancer, like heart disease (or, for, that matter, almost any other disease), probably results from a variety of causal factors acting in concert, but it has been estimated that the portion of total cancer in the United States that is significantly related to diet is 60% for women and 40% for men. Cancer is a major killer disease worldwide. Evidence suggest, that countries like India, Mexico and Africa have comparatively lower rate of Cancer incidence where as countries like Argentina and the United States have higher rate of cancer incidence. Countries like India and Mexico record lower levels of meat consumption, where as Argentina is the highest consumer of beef per person. Japanese, too, have lower incidence of cancer but those Japanese who move to the USA and whose consumption of meat increases, record higher rate of cancer. US Department of Health and Human Services (US DHHS) is on record with the statement, "A diet low in fiber and high in fat (read meat) with less consumption of fruits, vegetables and whole grain products, increases the risk of certain cancers. There is a growing consensus that cancer rates are lower in vegetarians, especially cancer of the breast and colon (non vegetarian diet specially that rich in animal fat has been found to be a risk factor for the occurrence of these cancers). Though surpassed in frequency by lung cancer, which is closely tied to smoking, colon cancer remains a major cause of death.

A meaty diet having high fat, high protein, low fiber content increase the risk of colon cancer for several reasons. Bacteria in the bowel modify dietary fat into carcinogenic substances that promote the growth of colon tumors. In addition, dietary fiber, moving through the colon, helps to dilute and bind the carcinogenic material and reduces its exposure to bowel wall. Vegetarians consume large amounts of fruits and vegetables which play a protective role against cancer. Carotene found in carrots, spinach, peaches and apricots and Vitamins found in broccoli, brussels sprouts, cabbages and oranges seem to reduce the risk of certain cancers.

Besides animal fat, barbecued meat and fish contain mutagens-substances that are known to induce cancer by damaging DNA in human cells. Broiling meat is also likely to form carcinogenic substances. Also, most animals raised for commercial or slaughtering purposes are given growth stimulants and hormones, many of which are believed to be cancer inducing.

Cancer of the prostate is less frequent in those whose diets are lower in fats and protein and richer in vegetables both of which are true of vegetarians. It is encouraging to think that the incidence of these three diseases, which together make up a large portion of the cancer occurring in world today, could be significantly reduced by the transition to a vegetarian diet.

Diabetes

Diabetes, another major health problem, is also less frequent in those who consume diets that emphasize rice, beans, and vegetables and fibrous food. A largely vegetarian diet has produced surprising improvements in many diabetics especially in those with the milder adult onset form of the disease. Such a diet has also been helpful for those who have other problems with blood sugar regulation, such as hypoglycemia. (obesity that is associated with non vegetarian diet is a major contributor to the development of diabetes of insulin resistance type)

Vegetarians also have lower incidences of a number of other common and trouble some disease, such as osteoporosis, diverticulosis and diverticulitis, gallstones and even constipation. What's more, most of the data available indicate that vegetarians tend to be slimmer and closer to desirable weights than non-vegetarians. This is important since obesity is an established risk factor for both heart disease and some forms of cancer, as well as being a common cause for concern in and of itself.

To sum up, it is beginning to appear that a vegetarian diet holds the potential for preventing disease on a scale that is for beyond what one might have imagined. Why would this be so? As research in the area becomes more sophisticated, it is clear that there are many faces to this question. As we shall see in subsequent sections of this book, a well balanced, largely, vegetarian diet, rich in whole grains, beans, vegetables and fruits corrects a number of serious defects in the body.

The Food Chain Effect

The food chain that prevails in nature is in the form of a pyramid. That is, at each progressive level there is concentration of the effects and more energy is required for the maintenance of higher order in the food chain. And this follows a 10% rule to make it simpler. For e.g. 100 kg of grains would be required to produce 10 kg of meat. (One can by themselves estimate that what a number of food shortage problem could be taken care if everyone turned vegetarian. For the amount of grain that would produce handful of meat would feed hundreds of people).

Also the food chain has a concentrating effect. Which means that each higher level the toxic substances concentrate in the body (for e.g. the grain treated with 10 mg of pesticide/ kg would get concentrated to 100mg/kg of flesh in the cow who ate it {and one can imagine well the concentration that would build up in a person consuming the same meat }).

Prion Diseases

Bovine Spongiform Encephalopathy (BSE), dubbed Mad Cow Disease because of the apparent mental torture cows display before death, is an always-fatal neuro-degenerative cattle disease caused by incredibly virulent and mysterious infectious proteins called prions. An outbreak in Great Britain had by early 1996 stricken around 160,000 cows. Circumstantial evidence pointed to the British practice of mixing the remains of sheep, including brains and bones, into cows' feed as the cause of the outbreak. This apparent species-to-species inoculation is what makes all forms of spongiform encephalopathy (known to affect other mammals as well) so alarming. Are cow-eating humans the next victims? At present, evidence pointed to a certain strain of Creutzfeldt-Jacob Disease (CJD) as being the human variant of spongiform encephalopathy. Grim predictions tell of up to 500,000 Britons a year falling to this disease due to their past consumption of BSE-infected cows. Prion-based diseases often have incubation periods in terms of decades, so the saga is sure to continue. In the meantime, since using the remains of dead animals in feed has been integral to agricultural operations in the US for years, BSE, or the chance of some future American version of it, is one more reason to think twice before biting into that char-broiled burger.

Foodborne Illness

"Meat and meat food products, and poultry and poultry products, contaminated with pathogenic bacteria are a leading cause of **foodborne illness.**" *Salmonellosis* is prevalent disease that occurs frequently in meat-eaters.

Plant Fiber and the Removal of Toxic Substances

With so many notes of alarm sounded by the news media about environmental toxins, it is easy to lose one's perspective to the matter. Actually, as we have seen, there are a number of frequently mentioned substances that at the present time pose no widespread or serious threat. Those that are still of considerable concern are primarily PCBs, lead, and mercury. A vegetarian diet may offer significant protection from all of them as can be deduced from what has been discussed above.

A diet made up predominantly of plant foods not only directly decrease one's intake of many toxic dose of red dye and other toxins but also reduces absorption of many toxins by actively binding them in the plant fiber.

Hence, some toxic substances in food can be held to a large extent by the plant fiber, are prevented from being absorbed in the body and carried out with the stool. Which toxic substance is absorbed probably depends on the particular fiber constituents present in the plant. This protective effect appears to be absent when the same chemicals are present in a highly refined diet, such as one made up predominantly of animal foods, white flour, sugar, fats, and oils. A vegetarian diet, rich in vegetable, fruits, grains, and beans and containing a variety of fiber types, should provide maximum protection. It has been shown, for example, that the pesticide level in the milk of nursing mothers was lower in those who were vegetarian.

Moreover a diet rich in high-fiber fruits, vegetables, grains, and beans also has a beneficial effect on the condition and functioning of the gastrointestinal tract. For all these reasons as long as the diet is properly designed so that deficiencies don't develop, the effects of a largely vegetarian diet should add up to significant improvements in health.

I Feel Better

There is a growing awareness that building health not only prevents untold suffering and expense but also has its more positive side. Being healthy feels better and permits one to do more, to be more active, and to enjoy life more fully. In order to contribute to the development of health of this sort, an optimal diet should not only prevent disease, it should increase one's strength and stamina.

Although today one might think of vegetarians as lean, light and airy even energetic, after a fashion they're apt to be considered a bit wanting in the area of strength and endurance. One who wishes to be strong eats meat or at least that's our collective image. The training tables of football teams groan under the weight of beef roasts and pork chops. To feed them otherwise would be courting defeat, right?

Wrong! Perhaps one of the best-kept secrets in the area of athletics is the surprising effects of a vegetarian diet on performance. Just after the turn of the century, experiments done in Europe and later confirmed in America produced results in exact contradiction to popular notions about athletic prowess and diet. The American studies, done at Yale in 1907, pille meat-eaters against vegetarians in a deep knee bending contest. Only one of the meat-eaters could reach the 1,000 mark, whereas six of those on the largely vegetarian diet were able to do so. In fact, two of the six vegetarians managed 2,000 repetitions each. A few similar tests have been done in recent decades looking at the more immediate effects of diet on endurance. In 1968, a Danish researcher found that for men on an average mixed diet, shifting to meat, milk, and eggs for three days cut endurance in half, whereas a purely vegetarian diet increased it by 50 %.

Although disappointingly little research has been done to follow up on these landmark studies, records set by vegetarians athletes are far out of proportion to their numbers. In 1956, a 17 year-old swimmer named Marray Rose became the world's youngest Olympic triple gold medal winner. He came back in 1960 to win further gold and silver medals, retaining his 400 meter title and becoming the first Olympic swimmer ever to do so. Later, he broke his own records and is considered one of the greatest swimmers of all time. He was a vegetarian. Other famous swimmers such as Johnny Weismuller, of Tarzan fame, have set multiple world records after following a vegetarian diet.

Not only swimmers but, vegetarian football players, basketball players, and even weightlifters have had distinguished careers. In the East these facts are not considered surprising. Observations of nature provide clues to the effects of diet. In the classic fight between the elephant and the lion, the elephant always prevails. Though more aggressive and ferocious, the carnivorous lion lacks both the strength and endurance of the vegetarian elephant. Long after the lion collapses in exhaustion the elephant stands alert and ready to continue.

A well-designed vegetarian diet not only increases strength and endurance, it also has been felt to clear the head. Many persons have spontaneously observed that a progressive decrease of meat in their diet has led to a greater clarity of consciousness. They value the relative alertness, calmness, and sense of equanimity that seem to accompany a meat-free diet. So far, little research has been done to explore such subjective observations. Nevertheless, it is intriguing to note for millennia the elimination of meat has been an important facet of many great spiritual traditions. It is almost a universal teaching that eliminating meat from the diet leads to a greater capacity for prayer, meditation, and self-awareness.

There is, moreover close correlation between cultivating health and expanding and sharpening awareness. The two pursuits go hand in hand because they work together so synergistically a healthier person is better able to be calm and alert because he's less distracted by illnesses and discomforts. A person who cultivates alertness and awareness is better able to understand his body, regulate it, and increase his level of health.

Skin

Compare this-vegetarian have lesser visit to doctor and the dentist, their skin is brighter and beautiful and their bodies are purer and cleaner in comparison to the meat-eaters.

Effect of Antibiotics

This is one such danger of eating meeting that is not easily known to the common man. The livestock reared for slaughtering purpose are given a large number of antibiotics to control the diseases they might be carrying. And over the period of time the slaughter animals are developing immune resistance to these antibiotics so that they remain diseased. Huge quantities of drugs also go into this function. In fact about 55% of total antibiotics used are fed to the livestock in the United States of America.

Another disease factor is that while or before being killed the animals secrete certain acids on account of fear and pain they suffer. This lead to development of disease-causing bacteria in the flesh of animals (the stress makes them more susceptible to infections). The end result is that the flesh is carrying diseases ever before it is processed and enters the refrigerator.

The arguments are endless and it would need a separate book to express them in detail. Let us now turn to the medicinal value of vegetables, fruits and other plant food.

Table 5.1: Deficiency, Diseases and Food Sources

S. No.	Deficient Food Element	Deficiency Diseases	Food Source
1.	Vitamin A	Loss of appetite, physical, weakness, Tendency to disease of eyes, ears, kidneys, lungs, skin, bladder, stomach and colon, pyorrhoea, anaemia. Slow mentality.	Whole milk, butter, cheese, egg yolk, yellow bhuta, yellow sweet potatoes, carrots and other naturally yellow and green coloured foods.
2.	Vitamin B	Indigestion of stomach and intestine, constipation, loss of weight and vigour, sub-normal temperature, paralysis of muscle groups, Neuritis, Glandular and endocrine disturbance including thyroid, adrenals, liver and pancreas.	Whole grain cereals, milk, butter-milk, green pear and legumes, dal, raw fruits, vegetables, honey, yeast, marmite. Part of group B is destroyed by cooking of those foods.
3.	Vitamin C	Loss of weight and physical weakness, Rapid heart and shallow rapid breathing, Bleeds easily. Low red blood Count. Teeth decay easily and become brittle, pyarrhoea, heart and blood vessel disease, scurvey.	Raw fruit especially oranges, lemons, tomatoes, guavas, leeches, mangoes, pineapples, chillies, sprouted grams, green leafy raw vegetables, potatoes, cabbage, milk. This Vitamin is destroyed by cooking.

Contd.

S. No.	*Deficient Food Element*	*Deficiency Diseases*	*Food Source*
4.	Vitamin D	Unstable nervous system. Low resistance to tuberculosis and other infections. Deformed bones, rickets.	Whole milk, few foods contain this vitamin, but it may be secured by daily exposing some part of the skin to direct sunlight.
5.	Vitamin E	Anaemia due to inability to digest the food iron. Failure of placental function thus affects child-birth.	Whole grain cereals, milk, green vegetables and raw fruits.
6.	Organic salts, Sodium	Diabetes, disturbed bile secretion. Flatulence with indigestion, constipation. Sodium is necessary to render lime and magnesia soluble for assimilation. Elimination of carbonic acid is facilitated by sodium in the blood.	Raw fruits and vegetables.
7.	Potassium	Defective growth with impaired glycogen function of the liver. Low red blood cell formation. Spleen function impaired. Low nerve energy.	Vegetables and cereals. Muscle tissue.

Contd.

S. No.	Deficient Food Element	Deficiency Diseases	Food Source
8.	Calcium and Magnesium	In nature calcium is always accompanied by magnesium. A large number of diseases of Childhood involving tissue changes and development are due to deficiency of these combined elements Abnormal intra-uterene development and difficult pattunition. Softering of bones (magnesium)	Fruit, vegetables and cereals. The green leaves contain relatively more calcium, while the seeds contain relatively more magnesium Nuts, milk.
9.	Iron	About 75 grains of iron in the human body. It enters into the human body. It enters into the most complicated compound found in the human organism. Good blood with all its vital consequences can only be formed with the presence of organic iron compounds.	Green leafy vegetables, onions, radishes, carrots, straberries, tomatoes, dates, apples, figs, cocoanut, walnuts. Bran of rice and wheat, Pulses, Yolk of egg, milk.

Therapeutic Value of Vegetarian Food

That vegetarian food is healthier and less prone to diseases for its consumers in comparison to meat-eater is now clear. But it goes much further and acts as medicine is something that needs a detailed study. In fact fruits, vegetables, seeds, spices etc. have their own medicinal value. Let us take them up in some detail one by one. First of all let us find out how different fruits act as curing agent s or medicine for our body.

Fruits

Apple-apple provides great nutrition and has high therapeutic value. The apple has 'malic acid' in it which is good for intestines, liver and brain. This fruit is full of vitamins and minerals including phosphorus. Apple is known to give strength to heart, improves eyesight, enhances memory, is good for patient of skin disease, mental disease, arthritis, breathing troubles and is a good sex tonic. It is a rejuvenating fruit. Doctors recommended in diseases like typhoid, hypertension, insomnia, gum swelling, liver related diseases, constipation, warts malaria, and several other ailments. It is not for nothing that it is said, "An apple a day, keeps doctor away."

Orange-Orange is a cool, soothing fruit. It has vitamin C, in it in ample quantity. Regular consumption of this fruit helps a person fulfill his vitamin C needs. Orange is considered a blood purifier. Typhoid, constipation, peptic ulcers chest diseases etc. are some ailments where consumption of this fruits helps. In jaundice also, consumption of orange is helpful. Beri-Beri, scurvy, joint pains are some other diseases in which juice of oranges helps the process of cure.

Mausambi-This fruit is extremely important as it is supposed to be elixir when eaten at the time of hunger. It is the permanent solution of sporadic cold and cough and is a rich source of vitamin C. Typhoid, asthma, heart disease are some diseases in which it helps greatly.

Mango-The nature of mango is hot so before eating it must be kept in cool water or refrigerator. The medicinal value of mango as well as cosmetic value separates it from other fruits. Eating mango regularly not only enhances physical and mental capability but also it improves aesthetic capability. As mango is a seasonal fruit, in one season one can store the required vitamins and minerals for one complete year. Juice of mango, if used at regularly brings power and removes feebleness of the body. Its use invigorates nervous system and rejuvenate the latent power of human being. "It is helpful in curing xerophthalmia and night blindness; simultaneously it enhances the resisting capacity. It contains more vitamin A than found in other indigenous fruits. It also contains vitamins B and C. Its vitamin potential keeps away the disease like Tuberculosis, Marasmus, Dysentery, Cholera etc. It strengthens the digestive system and keeps the people away from many liver related minor ailments". Raw mango is used in the case of sunstroke or it can be said that it works as panacea for sunstrokes. Eating mango produces blood in the body from which people feel more energetic and enthusiastic. It also removes the heart diseases and diseases related to kidney. It cures constipation and balances the habitual practices.

Grapes-Therapeutic value of grapes when known amazes one and all. It is useful in many maladies which have no cure in other therapies. The most deadly disease, cancer is helped by regular use of grapes. It is given in the form of juice to the patients suffering from Appendicitis, cancer, Pyorrhea, Asthma etc. It is helpful in the disease of Arthritis. It should be eaten in the morning to cure cough and cold. If blood comes out from mouth while spiting, grapes should be eaten. It's use normalizes the palpitation of heart. It is also useful in the case of restlessness. Small pox is also cured by eating grapes. It works as a tonic for not only children but also adolescences, teenagers and adults.

Banana-Banana contributes in controlling the diseases like gastritis, colitis, gastric ulcer, Typhoid etc. Banana is helpful in curing all kinds of swelling. Sodium is found in little quantity whereas potassium is found in ample quantity in it which helps in reducing the swelling. Vitamin C, riboflavin, and Thiamin is also found in banana. It lacks cholesterol and does not enhance the quantity of fat in the body.. Banana mixed in milk in form of shake is recommended for beautiful skin and regular bowel movement.

Pineapple-it is has wormicide qualities. In has similar to pepsin, Bromemilence which helps in digestion. it reduces blood pressure, cures cough and helps in Asthma etc. When tonsil develops or the throat swells, pine apple consumption is very much advantageous. It is helpful in diphtheria and keeps the throat clean, cures restlessness, lessens thirst and strengthens the body. It is also useful in strengthening mental power and keeps the belly cool.

Pomegranate-The medicinal value of pomegranate is enormous. It is useful in the diseases related to liver, dysentery, bellyache, obesity, cough and many more. Drying the leaves of pomegranate and making it powder mixed with rose water is used to remove the spots on skin. Due to the particular quality of being sour it enhances digestive power. It helps in treatment of bad odour out from mouth when water boiled with peels of pomegranate is consumed. If blood comes out from nostrils, consumption of its juice is recommended.

Guava-Guava is said to be the panacea for constipation and minor ailments related to liver. It throws out the itch and eczema. Not only the fruit but also its leaves are used as medicine. A hundred gram of guava has 299 to 450 milligram of vitamin C. it gives strength to heart and energy to body. The patients of malaria should be given guava.

Papaya-Papaya contains digestive acids which keeps the stomach clean. Papaya is generally eaten after meal. Papaya enhances the quantity of milk in lactating women. Taking papaya in boiled form helps cure dysentery. It removes constipation. The seed of papaya kills worms. Papaya should not be eaten by pregnant ladies.

Coconut-Coconut is helpful in many diseases. It removes headache. If blood comes out from nostrils, it can be helped by eating coconut regularly. It fulfils the requirement of water in body and checks dehydration. Taking the water of coconut is much too beneficial. It lessens the body temperature and is beneficial if consumed in summers. It also helps the patients of tuberculosis. Coconut water applied on scar marks reduces their intensity and also cleanses the spot of small pox. Common diseases related to eye are cured by regular use of coconut.

Carrot-Carrot is nicknamed as the apple of the poor as it contains lot of nutrients. It has life saving quality. It contains mainly vitamin A but vitamin B, C, D, E, G and K are also found in it. Its juice contains sodium, potassium, calcium, magnesium and iron and is useful in many diseases like tonsillitis dysentery, anemia, acidity, ulcer etc as also in returning the vitality of patients who have long been sufferer of diseases. It contains all elements of balanced diet. Black carrot cures Acidosis and is useful in case of skin diseases like itch and eczema. Liver diseases can also be cured by eating or taking juice of carrot. Due to vitamin A which is amply found in carrot it cures night blindness and diseases related to eyes. In case of marasmus, juice of carrot is efficacious. Its regular consumption strengthens teeth and brings shine. In winter season dryness of skin is common, which can be removed by eating carrot.

Myrobalan-Myrobalans is said to have power to cure all kinds of diseases. It gives youthfulness and reduces the palpitation of heart. It is rich in vitamin C; Human body daily requires 50 milligram of vitamin C which is found in the 1.6 ounce of the juice of myrobalan. One myrobalan has power equal to two oranges. It is useful in reducing blood pressure. It brings shine to the teeth. Stammering of children can be cured by chewing fresh myrobalan. It also cures diabetes and kills worms. For increasing the memory power, eating myrobalan is the best means. It enhances eyesight. Its medicinal value compared with its availability keeps it at apex. It improves the digestive system of the body.

Syzygium Cuminii : This fruit is also helpful in curing many diseases. It removes cough and diabetes. It brings hunger and keeps bowels clean. It also helps in curing damaged kidneys and keeps throat clean.

Tamarind: On being affected by sunstroke consumption of juice of tamarind is effective. It also removes itch and eczema. In summers, if one is affected with fever, one should be given drink made of tamarind.

Lemon: Lemon is said to be anti-toxin fruit which is found and used in all the seasons. Squeezing the lemon in one glass of boiling water and then drinking gives a lot of energy. It enhances eye sight and is a rich source of Vitamin 'C'. Use of lemon cures anemia, constipation, dysentery, blue, yellow fever etc. It also cures obesity. If it is taken daily, early in the morning empty stomach, it brings, slimness to body. It strengthens teeth and removes odour from the mouth. While traveling taking lemon is advantageous. Mountaineer use lemon while mountaineering. It removes the weakness of heart and balances blood pressure. In case of Arthritis also taking lemon is beneficial. It removes spots on skin. Using it on skin brings fairness.

Vegetable

Potato: This king of vegetables is hot and dry in nature. It is complete food in its own as it is a rich source of starch and of Calcium, iron, vitamin B and phosphorous. It maintains long life. People suffering from Beri-Beri can experiment with potato. Regular consumption cures from Beri-Beri and vitamin C found in potato cures scurvy. In scurvy blood comes out through hair follicles and later causes hyperkeratosis. Potato liberates from a lot of diseases like heart burn, acidity gout, arthritis, rheumatism, lumbago, renal stone, erysipelas etc. In dry potato 8.5% protein is found. To improve the colour of skin its peel is prevalently used. The patient of kidney should also eat potatoes in different forms. In potatoes, magnesium is found which lowers blood pressure. The nature of potato is basic so it lessens acidity.

Onion: Though hot and dry in nature it has many medicinal qualities. It removes insomnia and if regularly used, enhances the eyesight, cures pterigium and cataract. In case of sunstroke, onion is beneficial. Hiccough gets removed by the use of onion. It cures constipation and brings hunger. The adverse affect caused by changed place and atmosphere is removed by eating onion. It also cures dyspepsia, dysentery and diarrhea. Its paste is used for blackening the hair. Usage of juice of onion on warts, they are said to disappear. It also enhances the quantity of milk in women. All kinds of headaches can be removed by using onion. Raw onion, on being eaten kills injurious bacteria of mouth. In the paralysis also use of onion is effective. It removes dropsy.

Tomato : Tomato is neither hot nor cold in nature according to ayurveda. The author of Diseases and Diet has written that as much vitamin A, B and C is found in tomato is not found in orange. It is more beneficial than grapes or oranges. Each 100 gm of tomato contains 0.9 gm protein, 0.2 gm fat, 3.6 gm carbohydrate and other nutrients. Apart from this lime and iron are also found in tomato. It enhances the power of digestive system. It cleans intestines. It is beneficial in case of appendicitis, kills worms, reduces blood pressure and obesity, helps in skin diseases, reduces weakness and brings energy and enthusiasm. In the case of high fever tomato should be taken as it reduces the body temperature. It also enhances the growth of child. I also prove to be beneficial in case of marasmus.

Garlic : It has a lot of medicinal qualities. In several kinds of diseases it proves to be panacea. Its qualities can be summarized in following points.

1. It awakens hunger.
2. It bring shine on the face.
3. It saves from skin diseases.
4. It enhances blood and power.
5. It is beneficial in whooping cough, malaria, constipation, fever and swelling.
6. It removes the odouous smell of mouth.
7. It saves from tuberculosis.

Apart from these qualities, it has tremendous power to keep many diseases away. In case of diphtheria, hysteria, dropsy, cholera using garlic is beneficial. If one has become bald, using the juice of garlic is beneficial.

Radish: Its nature is hot as well as cold. Easy availability of radish is boon to people. It keeps many diseases away. Soup of radish is said to check formation of gall stone. In case of less formation of urine, radish usage is beneficial. Diseases related to kidney can be checked by regularly eating radish. It keeps the throat clear and cures hiccough. Tuberculosis, jaundice and acidity are the diseases which can be removed by the regular use of radish. In using its paste upon itch, it gets cured after some days.

Cabbage: Drinking the soup of cabbage cures the patient of peptic ulcer. Its leaves, if eaten regularly remove constipation. It also smokes out the negative elements from the body. In case of cancer, daily intake of its juice in the morning is beneficial. It also cures insomnia and colitis.

Cucumber: In cucumber silicon and Sulphur is found amply, which helps increase hair. If uric acid is increased, juice of cucumber should be taken. A rich source of Potassium it balances high and low blood pressure. It smoothens skin and brings shine on the face. It cleanses the spots on skin.

Spinach: All the qualities of a good vegetable are found in spinach. In it iron, vitamin A, B and C, and calcium are found amply. It is the best cure for pyorrhea. It enhances eyesight and removes constipation and keeps the many minor diseases related to intestines away. It also cleanses the blood.

Momordica Charantia: hot in nature, it is more beneficial if it mixed with ghee. It is more useful for the patients of paralysis and plays pivotal role in curing many diseases. It is called the safi of intestinal diseases and many liver related diseases get cured by the regular usage of it. In case of cholera and dropsy also, it is much beneficial.

Lady's finger: It is full of nutrients. A rich source of vitamin B complex, protein is also found in good quantity. Iodine, potassium, and phosphorus are amply found. It also has anti-inflammatory nature. In case of dysentery it is more beneficial.

Brinjal: It is hot and dry in nature, gives power to heart and cures acidity. If sweat comes out from hand and foot, its juice is beneficial.

Turnip: Turnip is useful for chilblains. The patients of diabetes should consume turnip daily. In the diseases of teeth and gum in the swelling of fingers, turnip should be given. Patients of Asthma should also be given the soup of turnip as also patient of cough and cold.

Other Plants Products

Green Gram: In case of fever, green gram is the best food. It should be taken with its peel. Green gram is also beneficial for the eye related diseases. It gives energy instantly. Those patients who are prohibited to be given solid food, should be given green gram. It removes constipation is beneficial in cases of itch and eczema.

Phaseolus Radiatus: It is useful for the patients of arthritis, paralysis and asthma. It has energy giving quality. It can be taken in any form. It removes hiccoughs. If blood comes out from nostrils, paste of phaseolus should be applied on forehead. It also removes baldness. In cases of leukoderma, application of its paste is beneficial. It is much beneficial for heart and mind as it provides mental as well as physical power.

Cajanus Cajan: It is hot in nature and saves from itch and eczema. Sweat can be checked by applying its paste on the body.

Black Gram: Black gram is eaten in many forms. But the sprouted black gram is the most beneficial of all. It gives power to body and mind. In case of dropsy, water of black gram is useful. It lessens the quantity of water in the dropsy. Vitamin C is abundant in sprouted black gram. It is highly proteinaceous. It helps in weight reduction and also cures constipation. In cases of diseases related tob respiratory system it is said to act beneficially.

For curing different ailments there are different methods of taking black gram, for example, for headache, powder of gram is mixed with ghee and then eaten. It is effective in jaundice, cough, polyuria and leucorrhoea. It is useful for the patients of heart disease. Its powder also enhances skin colour.

Lens esculentus: Its nature is hot and enhances concentration of blood. Its pulse is useful in many diseases related to liver. It helps clear away pimples from the face.

Wheat : Wheat in many form is effective and efficacious in many diseases. It keeps the digestive system normal. Sprouted wheat is eaten to keep the body fit. Its paste is used to cure itch and eczema. The plant of wheat has much more qualities. Wheat grass juice is said to be green blood. It is said that it looks after human blood to a great extent. It also cures cancer. Dr. Wigmor says that there is no any disease which cannot be cured by wheat. It removes the weakness of old age. For old age it is said to be panacea. A lot of doctors have suggested its use. From the usage of green grass the possibility of blood pressure, heart disease, paralysis and polio becomes slim. It enhances physical and mental growth and increases memory power. It awakens hunger and improves eye sight. It is experimented that if green grass of wheat is kept in water to be purified, bacteria and other impurities in water sticks to the leaves and water becomes purer. It also strengthens teeth and helps in cases of skin diseases. Juice of green grass should be consumed afresh. It also blackens hair.

Maize: Maize is a great source of carbohydrate. It is useful in cases of cough, whooping cough. Oil of maize enhances physical power.

Date: Taking two dates while going to sleep cleans voice, balances blood circulation, helps in cases of paralysis and body ache and when consumed with milk, helps in calcium uptake by body thus preventing diseases due to calcium deficiency.

Almond: Lime, phosphorus and iron are found amply in almond. If burning sensation is experienced while urinating five almonds, with elaichi, and sugar according to taste mixed with water taken twice daily helps. It also enhances memory power and is helpful in all kinds of diseases related to eye. Its ash is used for cleaning teeth.

Stammering gets cured if almond is taken with butter. It lessens the weakness of the body. In case of jaundice also, it is useful.

Walnut: It brings youthfulness even in old age if eaten regularly. It kills worms and rejuvenates body and mind. It is also effective in tuberculosis.

Basil (Tulsi) : Basil brings coolness to mind, enhances memory power and is a prophylaxis against malaria. It removes the negative elements of throat and loosens phlegm that gets accumulated in throat. In many diseases such as pneumonia, cough, headache, cholera, dysentery, liver related diseases etc., basil is useful. In tooth ache it reduces pain when consumed. If blood comes out from nostrils, juice of bastil should be dropped (4 drops) in the nostrils. It kills worms and awakens hunger and helps in digestion. In belly ache, equal quantity of the juice of ginger and basil heated together should be taken. It proves to be very helpful. Dysentery, leukoderma, Asthma are other diseases in which it finds its use. Leaves of basil remove all kinds of odorous smell.

Ginger: Ginger is hot in nature and is used in curing general diseases. It removes the odorous smell of mouth as also headaches. In case of cough, 30 gm of ginger and mixed with 30 gm of honey should be taken daily. It has proved to be very effective. In paralysis, ginger mixed with phaseolus radiatus should be consumed. In case of joint pain, ginger is effective. Dysmenorrhoea and tinnitus are cured by use of ginger. It also removes hoarseness.

Cardamom: Its nature is neither hot nor cool. It removes the smell of mouth and burning sensation while urinating. In case of belly ache and headache cardamom is effective. According to the survey of Elaichi Board, cardamom has capacity to remove any kind of pain.

Cinnamon: Chewing cinnamon cures stammering and strengthens digestive system. It is also used in cases of dysentery.

Plantago Ovata: It removes constipation and is very useful in amoebic dysentery. It checks mucus and removes burning sensation while urinating. In case of asthma also, it is effective. It removes even twenty-thirty year old asthma if it is regularly taken for six months to two years.

Tea: Tea is the medicine from plant family ideal for people living in cold climate. Tea increases blood pressure and excites nervous system. It removes tiredness and helps in cough, headache or fever due to cold. In sinusitis, tea consumption is injurious. Tea contains polyphenol which kills the organism of dysentery.

Coffee: coffee contains caffeine which excites the sensory cortex of brain and lessens pain. If there has been bout of asthma, coffee without milk should be taken. It helps in digestion and when taken after meal makes one feel light and happy. It also reduces the adverse affect of wine and opium.

Mustard Oil: it is used primarily for massaging skin especially during winters and relieves headaches by being massaged on the affected parts. Cough is said to be cured by applying mustard oil on nose. If any part of body has got burnt, mustard oil should be applied on that part of body.

Sesamum Indicum: It is the powerful food of winter season, is beneficial in skin diseases, constipation, cough, dandruff and by virtue of calcium content strengthens bone and teeth. Vitamin B complex is also found in it. It removes mental illness and hypertension and is also beneficial in rheumatism.

Castor Oil: It removes constipation if it is taken (two tea spoonful) while sleeping. It can be taken with hot milk or water. It is also beneficial in pyorrhea. Castor oil enhances beauty and removes pimples and is also helpful in arthritis.

Clove: Clove is beneficial in many diseases. It removes acidity. Though, manner of taking clove in different diseases is different. It cures many eye related diseases. It is also beneficial in tuberculosis and should be given with honey on appearance of measles. Whooping cough, typhoid fever, nausea etc are also cured by clove.

Aniseed: Aniseed enhances memory power and brings coolness to mind, quickens digestion, cures dysentery and removes bellyache. In case of high fever, its water is beneficial.

Turmeric: Turmeric is used to cure many diseases such as chilblain. Used in teeth disorders, its method of usage varies from disease to disease. Regular use of turmeric is effective in case of fractured bone. It cures acidity, eye-related diseases, Small pox, cough, asthma, expectoration, sciatica etc.

Rice: Rice is the main source of carbohydrate. Its nature is cold. In case of dysentry, eating rice is beneficial. Consuming rice for long span of time lessens the quantity of Cholesterol in the body. It also normalizes blood pressure. Before sunrise, taking a little quantity of rice thereafter drinking water strengthens the liver.

Asafoetida:. It lessens headache and bellyache, kills worms and awakens hunger which is ultimately helpful for liver. It keeps blood pressure low, cures hysteria, Urticaria, gives strength to heart and checks freezing of blood in the body. In homeopathy, many medicines are made from asafoetida. It also checks the effect of toxin in the body.

Black Pepper: It is used in weakness, in cases of dysentery, cough, headache, acidity, worms, itch and eczema. In cleaning the throat its use is beneficial. It also makes the voice sweet.

Capsicum Annuum: The nutrients which are found in capsicum annuum are given in table below.

Table 5.2 : Nutrients in Capsicum Annuum

Nutrients	*Indian Capsicum annum*	*Dried Capsicum annum (long)*	*Capsicum*
Protein (gm)	2.9	-	1.3
Carbohydrate (gm)	3.0	31.6	4.3
Calcium (ml. gm)	30.0	160.0	30.0
Phosphorus (ml. gm)	80.0	370.0	-
Carotene (ml. gm)	17.5	34.5	42.7
Vitamin C (ml. gm)	111.0	50.0	1.38

In capsicum annuum, Vitamin A and Vitamin C are found amply. It ignites the enzymes which help in digestion.

Coriander: being cold in nature it saves from sunstroke. It keeps many diseases away in summer season. It removes the pain of throat. If there be burning sensation in hand and feet it should be ground with sugar and then taken four times a day.

It lessens the palpitation of heart. In belly ache sharbat made from coriander is useful. Its juice brings hunger and is helpful in headache. In case of insomnia, green coriander should be taken with sugar. It removes the mental weakness, enhances eyesight and cures malaria when taken with grinded ginger. It also removes constipation.

Betel Leaf: Betel leaf is cold in nature. It should be eaten after meal. In diseases related to kidney, chewing betel leaf is useful. In case of cold and cough, betel leaf with clove should be eaten. In pyorrhea also it is helpful.

Camphor: In teeth pain, camphor is very useful. It kills the bacteria of teeth. In pyorrhea, it should be applied on gums with ghee. It is also helpful in itch and eczema.

Azadik Rachta Indiaca: It cleanses the blood. The juice of its leaves is useful to cure itch, eczema and blood pressure. Its leaves kill worms. Consuming its leaves boiled with water helps to cure many diseases. Its oil is useful in many diseases an in curing skin diseases. In case of white spot on the body, paste of its leaves and seeds should be applied. In leprosy, constipation, worms, skin diseases, scar etc it finds its use.

Sugarcane: daily consumption of juice of sugarcane keeps the health sound. In whooping cough, a little bit of the juice of radish mixed with one glass of sugarcane juice is beneficial. It cleanses the blood and checks hiccoughs. In jaundice also juice of sugarcane is helpful. Sugarcane also helps in digestion.

Nutmeg: It digests the food quickly. It is beneficial for black spots on face when applied after being grinded with milk. Its use stops dysentery and lessens pain. It is also a cure for insomnia. Nutmeg rubbed with ghee and then applying on eyes brings sleep sooner.

Caraway: The main characteristic of caraway is that it is digestive and pain killer. It removes fever, weakness caused by fever and other old show fevers. In malaria its use is effective. From its digestive powder is made. After boiling it and then washing the face with it enhances beauty of the face. In case of acidity its use is effective. It also removes itch from the skin.

Pear: Pear strengthens heart, mind, intestine and liver and also removes constipation. It is harmful in fever especially in typhoid.

Thus, we find that vegetarian food products are not only healthy and nutritious but also carry great medicinal value.

The whole humanity has now realized it and worldwide movement towards vegetarianism, has become noticeable. Besides diseases mentioned above, vegetables are also great skin nourisher. Let us know which vegetarian items are good for skin and in what ways.

Vegetarian Food and our Skin

Leafy Greens: Leafy greens like methi, spinach, drumstick leaves are full of antioxidants. They are a great source of iron when eaten with Vitamin C rich foods. Such foods make the skin shiny.

Ripe Tomato : This skin-sensational food packs high levels of the antioxidant Vitamins A and C as well as skin cancer fighting chemicals. Vitamin C helps keep skin elastic and prevents bruising. Vitamin A aids in healing acne from the inside out by boasting resisting to infection.

Berries: They are a great source of polyphenols, antioxidant that are currently being studied for their anti-aging capabilities. A hefty handful of strawberries or just 2 to 3 amlas has all the antioxidants Vitamin C our body requires each day to reconstruct collagen, the scaffolding that keeps skin from drooping.

Melon: This colourful fruit is full of carotene-like compounds such as lycopene which reduce the deep down collagen damage that promotes wrinkles.

Carrots: Carrots are burning with betacarotene which our body turns into Vitamin A, for keeping dry, flaky skin at bay.

Smart eating will help to ward off skin problems and keep wrinkles at bay. One should avoid over consumption of saturated fats and sugar for they may gum up the capillaries that whisk nutrients to the skin, thereby contributing to saggy, inflexible skin and brown spots.

Medicinal Value of Milk

Milk is useful in cure of several ailments. It induces growth in small children. If a child is suffering from malnutrition, he can be cured by giving milk along with almond regularly. Regular consumption of milk enhances *eye-sight* and improves the *retention power of brain.*

Those having *acidity* are recommended to consume cold milk. *Skin-irritation* is cured by rubbing milk on the affected portion of skin before taking bath. In case something falls in the eye, two-three drops of milk put in the eye remove the foreign particle due to greasiness of milk. Some diseases related to urinary bladder are cured by consuming milk with jaggery. Several other ailment like constipation, dysentery, breathing troubles etc. are cured by taking milk along with different things like *Isbgol, spices, dry fruits,* etc.

Milk also stimulates the sexual desire in both men and women. It is strongly recommended by doctors of various branches of medicine to consume milk at night before going to bed. It not only stimulates the desire but also increases the staying power and strengthens semen in men.

Milk can also be used to enhance the beauty of skin. Applying milk on the face and body everyday, make the skin shiny and fair.

Medicinal Value of Milk Products

Curd: According to Gastroentologist expert of Bulgaria Prof. Tasho Tachev, the intestines can be saved from the side-effects of antibiotics if curd is consumed during the period when antibiotics are being taken.

Curd is also useful in ailment like high blood pressure, obesity and diseases related to kidneys. Regular consumption of curd is good for prevention of heart disease. It acts to limit the formation of cholesterol in blood. Consumption of milk with black pepper, saunf and sugar can help avoid sleeplessness. Occurrence of various kinds of cancers is also prevented by consuming curd.

Though curd is made out of milk but it has some qualities that are even more important than in milk.

Butter Milk: Also known as *Chhachh* or *Mattha,* butter milk is also an important milk derivation that has some medicinal value.

Consumption of buttermilk along with *ajwain* helps in keeping piles in check. It also controls formation of fat in body. This product also helps in disease like blood pressure, asthma, malaria-related liver disease, indigestion, etc.

Butter: Consumption of butter is helpful for patient of tuberculosis.

Ghee: Ghee helps remove black spots on face and scar marks. It improves memory; applcation on burns it helps cure them; good to control cough and cold. In case of snake bite, consumption of ghee in large quantity (100-125 gm) helps remove the venom.

Importance of Soybean

In recent years great interest has been evinced in the cultivation and the use of Soybean, mainly on account of its dietetic, Industrial and agricultural importance.

Dietetic Importance

The bean is very useful in the preparation of bread, biscuits, cakes, pastries, soups, omelets, sprouts, Indian dishes like pulav, dal, chevda, shev, bhajias and many other tasty dishes-Indian, European, Chinese, and Japanese. Soybean is especially interesting to vegetarians on account of its richness in protein, fat, carbohydrates, mineral, salt and vitamins.

Analysis of Soybean shows that its protein is of a high biological value and resembles protein in meat, fish and eggs. The analysis, biochemical researches and feeding tests on rats show that Soybean contains three vitamins A, B and D; when it is sprouted it contains vitamin C also. Soybean is rich in the mineral salts of calcium, sodium, manganese and phosphorus in appreciable quantities.

Soybean milk resembles cow's milk in its properties and has been the main source of life for centuries in the oriental countries, namely, China, Korea and Japan.

Industrial Importance of Soybean

Soybean is very useful on account of its industrial importance. It is used in the manufacture of lard, margarine, vegetable, ghee; also used in the manufacture of paints, varnishes, linoleum, water proof goods, paper umbrellas, printing inks, celluloid goods, glycerin, rubber substitutes, fire works and explosives.

The oil of Soyabean contains lecithin and vitamin A and resembles butter in its properties. When there is a shortage of olive oil in the world markets Soyabean is substituted for it.

It is an edible oil and is used by the people of china and Japan for cooking purposes. It is also used in lubricating machinery.

Agricultural Importance

Every part of Soyabean is useful. The forage is made into green manure, hay, and ensilage and soiling. The milch cattle give more milk when they are given Soyabean feed. In America, it was found that hogs when provided with Soyabean feed, had put on more weight.

After the oil has been extracted the resulting residue called cake or meal is very rich in protein and mineral salts and is very valuable as fertilizer for the soil, as a feed for the livestock animals and as flour for human food.

Soyabean improves the soil on which it is grown like other leguminous plants; it takes its Nitrogen from the air, and not from the soil. It transfers the Nitrogen thus taken from the air into the soil, making it rich and fertile. It serves as a rotation crop. It improves the agriculture of the country and gives food to millions. It supplies fodder to the cattle and manures to the fields. Soyabean is comparatively cheap and gives the maximum amount of energy at minimum cost.

America was the first country to recognize the importance of this plant and now Soyabean is cultivated all over the States of America. Soyabean and Soyabean flour can be had in every grocer's shop in America.

During recent years some European countries have taken to the cultivation of Soyabean. They are England, France, Italy, Germany, Austria, Switzerland and the Balkan states.

In the "Five years Plan" Russia has set aside vast tracts of land for the cultivation of Soyabean. There is a Soyabean Research Institute at Moscow. An exhibition of Soyabean food was held where 300 varieties of Soyabean dishes were prepared including cake, pastry, salads, biscuits, chocolates, toffee, tea, coffee, cutlet, meat substitutes, soup etc. It was served to the representatives of trade-unions, factories, engineers, soviet Press and the Red Army. The food was unanimously pronounced to be excellent.

In Italy Signor Mussolini has founded a Soya Research Institute to investigate into the possibilities of its introduction in that country. He has ordered a study of Soyabean food values. It is said that in Italy Soyabean flour is added to the rations of the armies and breads containing 15 to 20 per cent of Soya flour are made by the order of the Italian Government.

Medical Importance

Soya flour is of great importance in diabetic dietary. Its starchy contents being quite negligible and its saccharides low, it is most suited to diabetic patients. Its carbohydrates are mainly such as to give energy without being provocative to the appearance of the sugar in the urine. This is why medical practitioners prescribe Soyabean flour in the diabetic dietary. Dr. Jozef Szanto in his pamphlet on "Soyabean flour in the treatment of diabetes" writes that he used to give Soya flour to the diabetic patients under his charge in his sanitarium with great success.

It is recognized by the medical profession that phosphates are very important for the brain cells and nerves. Soyabean contains abundance of phosphates so that it can be used with advantage, for the cure of nervous diseases. Some medical authorities have used them for the cure of rickets, pulmonary diseases, anemia etc. with great success. Dr. Levin of the Rockfeller Institute of New York found in it another brain building substance called Cephalin.

Soyabean is alkalizing in its effects

Meat, fish, eggs, cereals and pulses produce acidity in blood tissues while Soyabean is alkalizing in its effects. Studies made by Osborne at Barbara's Hospital show that after a meal of Soyabean the alkalinity of the blood increased. Soyabean food neutralizes the acidity in the blood. It is very important from the medical point of view as the normal alkaline state is the state of highest health and physiological functioning, while the acid state is pathological condition.

Protein from meat increases the amount of uric acid in the system and thus creates rheumatism, kidney troubles and gout. Protein from Soyabean on the other hand neutralizes uric acid and does not produce any disease. It is said that gout is unknown in China. Soyabean milk as well as its flour is used in food for invalids and infants, like Nestle's food.

Longevity and Soyabean

In China and Japan, Buddhist monks never eat meat. Protein in their dietary is supplied by Soyabean and its products. It is statistically proved that they are the longest lived people in those countries.

The lecithin content of Soyabean is high and so it makes a fair substitute for eggs. The medical science is unanimous in recognizing the fact that lecithin is quite essential for building up the nervous system.

Hence we have seen that vegetarian diet is not only nutritive but also has medicinal qualities.

6

Special Aspects of Vegetarianism

I this chapter we are going to discuss some practices that are integrated with vegetarianism in inseparable manner.

Milk

Milk : The Complete Food

Nature has designed milk in such a way that it provides complete nutrition to the new born of the mammalian species. It contains all that is necessary for growth and development in the tender years. The importance of milk as nutrition is hence indisputable and incomparable.

'Lacto' of term Lacto-vegetarianism indicate milk consuming vegetarians. Milk has been identified as the most nutrition food product since ancient times. Most of the societies insist on daily use of milk to maintain good health. In strictest sense of term 'vegetarianism' excludes all kinds of animal food and milk is surely a product that we get from animals. Such vegetarians are termed as vegans. Vegans argue that milk is required only in the yester years of life and not necessary in latter years and since it is derived from animals its use is totally prohibited. However we would discuss here milk as food and because of the above said controversy has been included in this section.

Milch Cattle

Milk of all animals is not suitable for human consumption. Mainly cow's, buffalo's and goat's milk is used for human consumption. Of these, cow and buffalo provide the bulk of milk to mankind. Camel's and elephant's milk is also occasionally used for therapeutic reasons. With consumption of milk and products rising rapidly, the dairy business has grown by leaps and bounds. The milch cattle has now become of great relevance to us today. Scientific technologies are being used to breed cattle of the best quality to increase procurement of milk. Slaughtering of such animal has come under criticism cause of not only the question of ethics but also for reasons of economics. The value of milk procured from them far exceeds the realization made through selling their flesh.

- This also adds another twist for meat-eaters. Those who consume beef often get the meat of sick and old cattle which have become worthless for yielding milk. This is particularly true in case of regions where strict vigilance is not kept on the food standards.

- In a country like India, cow is a sacred animal. People call it 'Gaumata' and revere as mother due to the good quality milk it provides. Killing of a cow is a sin in Hindu and other religions that practice non-violence.

Milk and Nutrition

India has a long standing culture in consumption of dairy products. Researchers had established long ago that children who are given boiled milk (unboiled milk can be a source of variety of infections especially bovine type of tuberculosis and transmission of some diseases from animal to man through) show improved health and growth compared to those not consuming milk. Stress is given on boiling of milk before consumption. Boiling inactivates certain-biologically active constituents of milk that are like to have adverse effect on the drinker of milk.

Milk is food designed to produce growth. Ayurvedic tradition recognizes the qualities of milk as a food and also its medicinal properties long since. Milk is *Kaphic* in Ayurvedic terms. It means that milk is suitable to match substance and matter of all the foods; it is more affective in matter producing since it is meant for children and to encourage growth in the infants. It is not only suitable for children but also for the adults. Its nutrition value can be gauged from the tables given below. Then three tables show the amount of nutrition provided by milk and milk products, different vegetables and meat products per 100 gram.

Milk is a wholesome nutrient and milk and milk products are capable of providing good nutrition to the body.

Ayurvedic precepts suggest that milk is best if taken in moderate amounts. Excessive quantities of milk are not easy to digest and can upset the stomach. As already mentioned, boiled milk should be preferred.

Pasteurization and boiling are the two methods to treat milk to make it safe before consumption. *Ayurveda* tradition do not encourage drinking of cold milk as it is likely to produce excessive mucus in the body. Consumption of milk in various other forms such as curd, Yoghurt, Cheese etc. is recommended and techniques to procure then products had been developed long-long ago.

Milk Products

Various food products are derived from milk by treating it different ways and by different methods. Such products are called milk products or dairy products. Some of them are briefly discussed below:

- *Curd:* Curd is made by coagulation of milk by adding acid to it or usually inoculating milk with a culture of specific microorganism (or using old curd to obtain the microorganism required). Warm milk is used to make curd. It takes a thickened form on being coagulated and has a sour taste. Curd is used as a food item and can be consumed either by adding salt, sugar or just like that. it is considered a cool (something that has a refreshing temperament) food item that helps in digestion of food and has a cooling effect on body. It is mostly taken with lunch but avoided with dinner.

- *Lassi,* a liquefied drink is prepared from curd and is prepared by stirring curd with some water and to it either salt or sugar is added. It is a rejuvenator especially in the months of summer and is usually avoided in rainy seasons and winter as per ayurvedic tradition.

- *Yoghurt:* Yoghurt is a semiliquid food made from fermented milk. It has its own fans and critics.

- *Homemade Cottage Cheese :* Popularly known as Paneer in India, cheese is a highly consumed variety of dairy product. It is prepared addition of lemon juice to milk. The effect of the acid of lemon juice added to the already boiled milk is not only to curdle it but to further the hydrolysis of the protein by breaking it down into constituent amino acids. The Cheese is processed by straining of the processed milk.

Paneer is considered a rich item and is widely used in preparation of a variety of Indian dishes.

The Cottage Cheese usually found in grocery stores is different from the homemade variety called Paneer. Cottage Cheese contains several additives and is not fresh. Paneer made by using lemon juice is fresher and healthier.

Preparation of cheese: To prepare a cup of cheese one needs half a gallon of milk. Bring it to boil and add some lemon juice. Stir them together and keep the milk simmering. Continue till the curd or thickened milk starts appearing. Allow the milk to boil for a few more seconds. Then leave it alone for some minutes. Now thickened cheese is formed and a liquid is seen separated from it. Strain off using a thin cloth. Squeeze out the cheese to bind it better and make tighter. Now it can be cut into cubes and added to vegetables dishes for cooking. The liquid that is separated is called 'whey' and is a nourishing substance used to make bread and also as beverage. It soothes the body and cleans the urinary tract.

- *Skimmed Milk:* Milk consumption is sometimes objected to, on grounds of its butterfat content. Butterfat increases the total fat levels in diet dramatically and also contains cholesterol. Nonfat or skimmed milk is offered as an alternative to milk. It is available in dry form as well as a variety of the regular milk in singly or doubly skimmed depending upon the fat content. However, butterfat plays a beneficial role in absorption of calcium in the body as well as various other vitamins.

- *Butter:* Butter is yet another milk derivative that finds extensive use in every day life. Most common use of butter include in making of sandwiches and as a cooking medium. In case of its use as a cooking medium, it is comparatively expensive and is not used freely at homes. But in restaurant it is frequently used and has its own class customers. Such places attract their customer with advertisement like 'cooked in butter', 'Butter-fried' etc.

Other cooking mediums that are used as a substitute to butter include saturated vegetable fats, vegetable oils, and animal fats such as lard. Animal fat is considered inappropriate by vegetarians and not used by them. Saturated vegetable fats like coconut oil, vanaspati ghee etc are preferred mediums because of their low cost. However food coked in butter has a special aroma and is widely preferred in cooking as stated above.

A moderate consumption of butter is advised due to its high content of saturated fat. (it carries with itself some quantity of water and milk as well until and unless fully processed)

Preparation of white butter: once the full cream milk is boiled it is allowed to cool down without disturbance. Malai (cream-a precipitate over the milk) is formed after some time and it is strained off to separate it from milk. Equal quantity of water is added to malai and is churned continuously either manually or in mixer for length of time till butter starts floating on top of it. It is then separated and used. The liquid that remains can be used as a drink by addition of salt to it and is cherished especially with meals in summers.

However, *ghee*, a product derived from butter finds more favor as a cooking medium.

- *Ghee or Clarified Butter*: As already pointed out, butter is not a pure fat; it also has water and milk solids in it. Ghee is derived from butter by boiling it.

Preparation of ghee: On boiling, ghee appears at the top of container in a clarified form while a sediment is formed at the bottom of the container. The sediment should not be scratched or stirred. It will spoil the ghee being formed. When the sediment turn brown the ghee is ready and boiling should be stopped. Boiling removes the water by evaporation. Ghee is poured off into a container. The sediment remains can be used in cooking of dishes or making of bread. The ghee or clarified butter freezes into solid form when kept in refrigerator. It also becomes solid even if kept in open in winter, butter liquefies on hot days.

Ghee is pure fat in saturated form and is the purest derivative from milk. Its consumption is advised only to judicious quantities because of its pure form.

Ghee is a favoured cooking medium in the world's two greatest culinary traditions-French and India. Classical French cooking relies heavily on clarified butter. According to *Ayurveda*, ghee has character of a preservative (this is reflected in the fact that many food items that are to be consumed over a long period of time are prepared in ghee) as well as a special capacity for picking up the medicinal benefits of seasonings and herbs and carrying them into body. Due to this reason several natural medicines made from herbs and spices are often prepared in a ghee base; it enhances their effect. Some medicines are consumed combined with the ghee in ayurvedic tradition.

It is found that when food cooked in ghee is compared with food cooked in vegetable oil after 24 hours of refrigeration, it retains greater freshness.

- *Other Milk Products* : The products derived from milk discussed above are mostly good from nutrition point of view. Besides, several other products are derived from milk that do not constitute any nutritional value but are consumed for taste. Such milk derivatives are quite soothing for our taste buds. The list of these products is quite extensive. Some of such products are discussed below.

(i) *Ice cream:* Popular world over, ice cream is gulped down the throat with great enthusiasm by people of all age groups. It is especially popular among children and teenagers and is a great money spinner. Ice cream has a large number of varieties. (Excessive consumption of ice cream leads to obesity, faster tooth decay and several other ailments.)

(ii) *Khoya*: Khoya is a traditional Indian product made by boiling the milk over with addition of sugar till its turns into solid. Khoya can be consumed directly. It also forms the base matter for various kinds of sweet products, dishes and preparation of Muglai gravies.

Preparation of khoya: milk is boiled and judicious quantity of sugar is added to it (it can be prepared even without addition of sugar). In a wide mouthed vessel it is then stirred slowly and continuously. After sometime milk will start loosing its water content and will become thickened. Caution should be taken not to stop stirring as this will spoil the preparation. In the end whole water content would evaporate and only dry solid will be left behind and is called khoya.

(iii) *Sweet Products* : Sweets like *burfi, rasagulla, peda, kalakand, milkcake* etc. are all milk derived products. These are quite popular among Indian masses.

(iv) *Kheer* : Kheer is made by boiling the rice in milk with addition of sugar.

- There are several other products-Custard, Chocolates, Milk shake etc; the list is endless. And thus we learn that milk is the food of the masses and essentially a vegetarian diet. The poor classes, who can't afford to consume milk directly, also make use of a great quantity of milk in the form of tea. In the Indian subcontinent tea is prepared by adding milk to it whereas in several other countries tea is prepared without milk.

Besides being a good nutrient and source of several popular food products, milk also has a great medicinal value. Milk and curd are used to cure various kinds of ailments

Fasting

Fasting and Religion

Fasting is a completely natural process which each one of us does at night while we sleep, and the next morning we break our fast with break fast. In India many Hindus, especially ladies practice regular fasting as part of their religious customs. Sometimes they fast once a week or on full moon days, if not a complete fast, they may take only fruits and other light food stuffs. Fasting is also an integral part of the Muslim faith, with day-light fasting during the holy month of Ramzan. In Buddhism and Christianity fasting is also of great importance. Christ and Buddha both fasted for 40 days before reaching enlightenment and starting their missions.

Saints of every order have used fasting with prayer or mediation. To reach higher spiritual states. Other people have used fasting solely as a practice to improve physical and mental health, while natural therapists have suggested that fasting is at the basis of curing many diseases. Fasting combined with yogic practices has been found to be very use full for digestive problems, helping to even eliminate them.

What is Fasting?

The, word, fasting comes from the old English word fasten meaning to fix or make firm. Under no circumstances does fasting mean starvation. In effect, the point where the body starts to starve because it has depleted its nutritional reserves is the end of the fast. From the outset it is important to realize the fasting stage one takes place so long as the body can support itself on the stored raves are depilated or are at a dangerously low level.

Fasting, like all other natural cures, is based on the principle that the body itself contains the most efficient waling agents. These agents are most effective when they are unhampered by the process of digestion and assimilation which tends to drain off much of the body's energies Fasting gives these systems a much needed rest and releases energy for the elimination of toxins and for restoring the body to health.

In the optimum state of health there is no need to fast, how ever. This is rarely the case. Most people continually over tax the body by eating too much, drinking too much and living in a continual state of tension. Bodily efficiency is continually impaired by the surplus of food which it is unable to use up or throw off. Fasting gives the body time forthright cleansing and expulsion of accumulated wastes and usage of what was extra in the body.

In the digestive tract there is a continuous build up of waste material such as undigested or partially digested food particles, bacteria and soon If a person habitually over eats or suffered from constipation this build up will be greatly increased. This is the breading ground for many more serious illness as well as general ill health. The simplest way to clean out the whole digestive system is to miss a few meals. When no food is being ingested the body can concentrate fully on what is already there. The build up of waste materials is more effectively expelled via the bowels, kidneys and skin, bringing about a marked purification of the blood. This in turn gives a wonderful feeling of lightness and freshness.

Many people are afraid to miss even one meal as they believe that this will weaken them. The fact is however, that modern man suffers mainly from disease of excess (obesity, diabetes, heart disease, etc.) He digs his grave with his teeth. life insurance statistics reveal that a trim body is conducive to a longer life span.

Fasting and Disease

Have you ever observed an animal, such as your pet dog or cat, when it is not feeling well? In most cases it will try to go some place where it will not be disturbed lie down and take complete rest. Even if your give it food it will refuse to eat. Human beings however find it very difficult to rest and recuperate, and for most fasting is nearly impossible, Many people think that energy comes from food and so tasty dishes are prepared for the sick person to induce him to eat. This attitude fails to take into account the fact that one of the first signs of sickness is a loss of appetite, a natural warning designed to help nature's repair work.

When bacteria invade the body the immune system is mobilized. All available energy is required to fight back and physical activity is avoided to redirect the energy. Eating requires a lot of metabolic energy and this energy must be kept in reserve for fighting the disease. Fasting speeds up the catabolic (break down) process which occurs in illness, there by helping to eliminate laxness. This appears to be the opposite view to that proposed by medical science which offers drugs and chemicals to reduce discomfort and suppress symptoms. However, if we allow the disease to complete its natural course it will be finished and the body will be purified. Many poisons are thrown via urine.

Fasting is more important for those who have been on a high meat diet. Those who only take animal products such as cheese, milk and eggs require less fasting. People on a pure vegetarian diet, fasting is not necessary, but it can be used occasionally in disease to rest the body, or to increase the digestive fire.

To claim that fasting is 'cure-all' no matter what the nature or duration of the disease, would be foolish. Fasting is a science and it must be practiced under expert guidance especially when utilized as a therapeutic technique. The age of the sufferer, the nature of the complaint (whether acute or chronic), and various other Considerations will all have to be taken into account, If an organ is structurally defective, fasting will not bring it back to its original state. However if there is any functional disorder, fasting is simple, direct and effective method of cure. It attacks disease at the roots by expelling poisons and also by increasing will power and inducing a relaxed, meditative state of mind which is very important in the removal of the tensions that cause disease.

Psychology of Fasting

Fasting must be practiced under the right circumstance and with the right frame of mind. If one is worried about toxins building up in the body or about becoming too fat, then fast will be ineffectual. There will be tension instead of complete rest and relaxation. Such fasting is not natural, arises out of desire or fear and throws the body's metabolism out of balance. It is better to call this short of process starvation instead at fasting.

You will know natively when it is the right time to fast. Something inside says it is better to miss a meal or two. Perhaps hunger is absent or you feel that you may be getting sick. When the body tells us 'No more food, please', it is nature's signal to fast.

Self imposed fasting can also be used as a meditative sadhana. If the hunger is great you can practice antar mouna and observe everything that goes on into the body and mind. Through this you will learn many things about your self and the importance of food in your life. You will see the psychological pull that hunger and taste exert as well as your habitual approaching attitude towards food. This is a method not only to discover the inner workings of the body and mind but also to develop mental strength and will power.

Fasting, when approached correctly, is very relaxing. As the body slows down the mind does also and this can be felt in the following ways;

Breathing is freer

There is greater ease of movement

'That tired feeling' disappears

Fullness and discomfort in the abdomen are soon replaced by lightness

Blood pressure is lowered.

How to Fast ?

Preparation for a fast is very important. It is not advisable to make an abrupt transition from your usual diet unless you are very ill. In this case all solid food should be eliminated from your diet and plenty of fluids consumed so as to flush the kidneys. If you will to prepare for the fast, first abstain form meat and heavy foods, then over the next few days switch over to alight fruit diet. After this you can commence the fast.

The following suggestions will help to make your fast more successful !

1. If possible, fasting should be undertaken during the warmer periods of the year. During cold weather, food is concerted into energy to keep the body warm. Fasting at this time makes the body more susceptible to cold.

2. Few people are aware of the benefits of fasting, so before you begin, make sure that your family and friends understand the basics of fasting and your goal. Fasting in the early stages may be difficult enough with hanging relatives, trying to force food down your throat. A positive, encouraging atmosphere amidst family and friends is most helpful. If you wish to fast for a long period of time and your surroundings are not suitable, we advise you an ashram or similar institution where fasting is regularly under taken with the aid of expert guidance. Most people are a little uncertain during their first attempt at fasting so it is essential that the environment be as congenial as possible.

3. The body itself is the most reliable indicator of how long the fast should be. This applies whether one is fasting for cure of disease or for general cleansing; the severity of the disease or for general cleansing; the severity of the disease determining the length of the fast. As the constitution of each of us is slightly different, the duration of fasting must suit each individual. Rely on what the body tells you rather than on the experience of others.

The duration of the fast depends largely on the purpose for which the fast is under taken for a general cleanout, 1 to 3 days per month is sufficient. If fasting is practiced once a week the benefits will greatly enhanced. For more specific purposes the standard duration is 3 days if one is without guidance. This is generally long enough to give the whole system a complete rest.

4. In a pure fast one should take only plain water, nothing else. It is good to drink plenty of water while fasting as this increases the natural process of purification. In a fast of longer than 2 days, one should

take water with a little lemon Juice (no sugar) 3 times daily to aid the cleansing process.

5. In a day's fast, feelings of weakness (if they occur) are largely psychological. Your mental attitude will make all the difference. People have been known to fast for many days and grow progressively stronger. Some people say that on a 1 day fast it is essential to maintain all normal activities, for if one rests all day 80% of the benefits will be lost due to lack of natural blood circulation. While fasting, most people experience a wonderful feeling of freshness and lightness, and many report that they can carry out their daily duties even more efficiently. The average person may wish to avoid strenuous physical activities on a fast of 3 days or longer. You must find your own middle way.

6. In prolonged fasts hunger sensations disappear after the first few days even though the hunger contractions of the stomach may persists. This is thought to be due to an adaptive process in the brain. Drinking water helps to relieve the desire for food, but never drink iced water. Also use bhujangini mudra to reduce hunger. Keep in mind that there is a difference between hunger and appetite. Hunger is the natural call of the body for food in order to maintain itself, while appetite is hunger of the mind.

7. It is beneficial to take an enema or to do basti or laghoo shankhaprakshalana on the day of fasting, or the day after, especially if there is no bowel movement. Do not use laxatives.

8. Bathe once or twice a day with cold or lukewarm water. Inner and outer cleanliness go hand in hand.

9. Keep yourself occupied mentally and do no think about food. One who fasts but spends the whole time waiting for the fast to be over is wasting his time and creating mental tension.

10. Fasting is not generally advised for reducing fat. The average dieter will fast for one day and then eat enough for three days the day after.

11. Look upon fasting as a spiritual practice form its physical benefits, fasting is a powerful method of developing will-power and self-discipline.

12. The important thing to remember in fasting is moderation. Never fast if the cravings of the body and mind become excessive, and don't fast if you do not feel/like it. Be open to the possibility of fasting and use it when the need arises. It is said in the *Bhagavad Gita* :

Yoga is not possible for he who eats too much, or for he who abstains too much from eating."

Breaking the Fast

There is a great tendency to over eat upon completion of the fast. Much care should be taken to ensure that a proper diet is followed. The method of breaking the fast will depend on the duration of the fast, but generally the first food taken should be liquid-fresh fruit juice or milk. This especially applies for fasts longer than 24 hours. Orange Juice diluted with water, taken every 2 hours is a popular way to break a fast. The first solid food to be taken should be something easy to digest, like melon or vegetable broth. Take only small amounts and chew each mouthful well.

The following diets are suggested after the liquid diet :

Fruit diet—preferably composed of chopped fresh fruits in season: apples and dates or peaches and dates, for example taken in small quantities every 2 or 3 hours. Milk diet—take a glass of milk every few hours as desired.

Gruel diet-boil a tablespoon of oatmeal or barley in a pint of water and add a pinch of salt or sugar. Take small amounts at first, slowly increase over a few days.

After breaking the fast, it is well to keep the following points in mind :

- Drink plenty of Water.
- Your stomach will have shrunk and will require less food so take care not to overeat.
- Don't over exercise for the first few days.

Partial Fast

Many people will find it impossible or impractical to complete a prolonged fast. For them we suggest a partial fast which can give many benefits although not to the same degree as a full fast. A partial fast involves restricting the diet to fruits, which cleanse the body by their accompanying laxative influence on the bowels and also supply the blood with needed minerals and vitamins. Here are some dietary suggestions for carrying out a partial fast:

1. 6 to 8 oranges a day—1 at a time every few hours.
2. 1 grape fruit every 3 or 4 hours.
3. ¼ pint of fresh fruit Juice every 3 hours, up to 6 times a day
4. 1 cupful of vegetable broth every 4 to 6 hours.

Should Children Fast?

Children often know instinctively when to fast. If you let the child miss a meal of even a day's food when he is sick, for example and doesn't want to eat, real hunger will soon appear. The child will naturally want food when the body requires it, especially if in between meals snacks are stopped and raw fruit is substituted for after dinner sweets. There are times when the instinctive wisdom of the infant or child in such matters may be for greater than many of us give credit for.

Fasting Sadhna

While fasting, yogic practices should be directed towards helping to eliminate the toxins of the body. The following techniques are particularly useful:

Hatha Yoga	:	Laghoo shankha prakshalana, Kunjal and neti, basti.
Asana	:	Pawanmuktasana, Vajrasana, Shavasana.
Pranayama	:	Bhramari, nadi shodhana, ujjayi;
Meditation	:	Yoga nidra, antar mouna.

Sprouting

In a mysterious way, there is locked up a life principle in every seed which can be turned loose and made perceptible by means of moisture and warmth. This is called sprouting. All grains, wheat, oats, rhye, barley, millet corn (maize), soyabeans, mong beans garvanzas (gram), foenugreek (metha dhana), alfatfa cooking are of immense nutritional value.

Food problem of the world will be solved and everyone will get best nutrition for perfect and sound health. Wanted: A vegetable that will grow in any climate, rivals meat in nutritive value, matures in three to five days, may be planted in any climate, any day of the year, requires neither soil nor sunshine, rivals tomatoes in vitamin C, has no waste in preparation but instead increases in nutritional value

Dr. Clive Mecay of Cornell was not just dreaming when he composed the above request. In fact, this utopian sounding wanted in concise and accurate description of immense qualities of most sprouts.

Research shows sprout in its first days of life is a veritable vitamin factory. Dr. Paw Burholder of Yale University (USA.) measured the following increase on the vitamin content of dry oats after only five days of sprouting:-

Niacin Acid	500%	Folic Acid	600%
Biontin	50%	Inositol	100%
Pantothenic Acid	200%	Thiamin (B1)	10%
Pyrodoxine (B_6)	500%	Riboflamin	135%

One cup of soybean sprouts contain an equal amount of Vitamin C as six glasses of orange juice. 100 gms of sprouted wheat has a greater nutritive value than the white bread obtained from a kilogram of wheat. The same is true of all the varieties of corns and pulses. These features cover the increase in B complex vitamins. The figures for Vitamin C show a similar Pattern. When we consider that virtually all sprouts (wheat, alfalta, lentils, garloanzas, mungbeans, etc.) develop in the same way we begin to understand the reason for their inestimable nutritive value.

While any grain or legume is suitable for sprouting, the simple and easily available alfalfa (Barseen) seed is considered to be the best of all as it contain all the known Vitamins including D,E,G,K,U,B complex and B8: besides potassium often called the Elixir of Life: phosphorus, which is considered a good brain food; and calcium, so essential for bones, teeth and general well-being. All sprouts contain Vitamin A, B and C equivalent to that found in fruits.

Besides the several elements, the sprouts contain, as explained above, they are filled with body building enzymes so essential for the digestion of food Enzymes enable the digestive organs to digest food properly, making its nutritional elements, especially the cell-building proteins available to the body. Dr. Earp Thomas, scientist of USA ascertained that lack of enzymes in the digestive system permits the toxins to build up in the colon which in results in the growth of ulcers tumors and malignant cancer.

The great importance of enzymes can be fully understood, if we compare the human body to an automobile. If the automobile engine is in good running condition and there is plenty of gasoline in the tank, but no spark to ignite the gasoline the car will not run. Enzymes, act as the spark that enables the digestive organs to turn the nutrients of the food we eat, into good, rich blood. The reason most people are tired is that there is a lack of Enzymes in their bodies. The food they eat cannot be utilized constructively, but is turned into toxins, or poison, which leads to sickness and disease. The value of sprouts is therefore greatly enhanced because of the presence of Enzymes which are so essential for health and longevity.

How to Sprout

All kinds of Grains, Cereals, legumes and other seeds such as, Wheat, Barley, oats, Maize, Bajra, Jawar, Gram moong, Mothh, methadana, Harhar, Malka Masur, Soyabeans, Peas, Alfalfa (Barseen), Sesame (til) and Groundnut can be sprouted in all seasons and all climates. For sprouting moisture and warmth is needed. The procedure for sprouting is very simple and can be followed by any one with the least difficulty. It is to be done as explained below:

(1) Clean the seeds very thoroughly and weed out any defective ones as well as some tiny pieces of hard substances.

(2) Then wash the seeds with water several time to ensure that no dirt remains.

(3) The seed should then be placed in some container of any kind preferably an earthen pot and soaked in water. Sufficient water should be put so that water is at least two to three inches above the seeds.

(4) The seeds should remain soaked in water from six to ten hours. Some harder seeds such as soybeans etc. will require more time while others will require less time. But ten hours is the maximum. It will be wrong to keep the seeds soaked in water for more time, as in that case these will begin to rot. Soaking in water is required for the seed to absorb sufficient moisture necessary for bringing it into life. This purpose is fully served in six to ten hours. The best thing will be to soak the seeds before going to bed and take them out in the morning.

(5) Take out the seeds soaked in water often six to ten hours and wash the same several times with running water.

(6) Now take a thick piece of cotton cloth. Size will be according to the quantity of material required for sprouting. Soaked seed should be put into this piece of cloth and loosely tied. This small, bundle may be hung with a peg or kept somewhere.

(7) After 10 to 24 hours the seed will germinate, and a tiny sprout will poke its way out and begin to grown. The time will vary according to season. In hot season, the germination takes less time than in cold season.

(8) During the period the seeds are kept tied up in the cloth it is to be observed that the cloth should not go dry. Water is to be sprinkled over it several times during the day especially in hot season to keep it always wet. Twice or thrice during the day the seeds are to be flushed with water to remove the slime that generally accumulates on the seed.

(9) Soybean or such like hard seeds require more time for sprouting. They also require more warmth. Such seeds after being tied up in a piece of cotton cloth should be fully covered with some thick woolen piece all around. Kept somewhere and heavy weight placed on it. Let it remain there for 10 or 15 hours and it will sprout. The time factor will be loss or more according to season.

(10) After the seed sprouts, it is ready for use. If the sprouting is allowed to continue for 60 to 72 hours its nutritional value increases tremendously as explained earlier.

(11) It will be useful to expose the sprouts to indirect sun for the last two hours of their growth before consuming, to make them green at the finish.

(12) After seeds are sprouted, before consuming, it will be advisable to place them in some flat plate and the defective and hard seeds that have not sprouted should be removed. This has to be necessarily done in the case of soybean, mooth and moong. If this is not done than while eating if any hard seed comes under your teeth, the whole taste is spoiled, little time therefore spent in weaning out will make you relish the sprouts.

(13) Whenever you wish to eat sprouts it will be good to wash and rinse them properly. After washing the sprouts those can be placed in a thick dry cloth and

worked up so as to remove the outward moisture. You will relish more when the sprouts have less moisture.

(14) After the seeds have sprouted those can be placed in a vessel, duly covered and kept in refrigerator. Those can remain for several days without spoiling. It must be noted that those should remain covered up. Those will not spoil even when kept outside but those must be washed as explained above and outer moisture removed.

(15) Each sprouted seed can be eaten separately but without the addition of salt or any other condiment. Sprouted seed has got its own delicious taste, why spoil it with some addition? However to create variety and taste, mix several sprouts such as moong. Mothh gram and alfalfa (Barseen); mix it with raisin (kishmish) which have been soaked in water for one or two hours and grated coconut. you can also add cashew nut or ground - nut soaked in water and its outer covering removed. This will make fine and tasty dish.

(16) For sprouting one can also make some container of wood with four or five apartments, side 4" to 5" high and on the base some kind of mesh with small holes is to be fixed up. On all the four corners and one in between on all the four sides 2" long legs should be fixed to this container. The idea is, whenever this container is placed on the flat surface excess water will drain off from the seeds kept for sprouting. The mesh can be of iron but it will be better if it is of brass or copper as that will not rust. Put some thick pieces of cotton cloth duly made wet underneath, place the seeds for sprouting over it and cover it them with another wet piece of cotton cloth. After every three or four hours you can put

water over this which will automatically drain. This will eliminate the process of tying up and hanging it with a peg etc.

Hence we have seen that with little effort we can increase the nutritional value of our food many times by simple method.

The Yogic View of Vegetarianism

It is assumed that vegetarianism is an integral part of yogic practice. This is only partially true however, for while yoga views vegetarianism as the most beneficial system of nutrition, it does not for an instant insist that practitioners of yoga become vegetarians. Although becoming vegetarian is preparation for higher forms of yoga, non-vegetarians are heartily accepted as practitioners of yoga. Yoga advises but does not preach vegetarianism.

Actually yogic practices in themselves have nothing whatsoever to do with diet, whether vegetarian or non-vegetarian. The aim of yoga is to expand the awareness and awaken the prana shakti which can sustain the body even in the absence of a so-called nutritious diet. By practicing yoga, both mental and physical health is improved, regardless of whether one is Vegetarian or non-Vegetarian.

At the same time yoga recognizes that food is as much necessity for the aspirant as mental, emotional and spiritual nourishment. In yoga a simple diet is used to fuel the physical body (annamaya Kosha), and hatha yoga to remove its impurities. Pranayama charges the vital energy body (pranamaya Kosha) while meditation develops the mental and psychic bodies (manomaya and vigyanamaya Koshas). As for as making food a path to higher consciousness, however no diet on its own has yet succeeded and the yogic diet is no exception.

Many people are surprised to find that there is no fixed yogic diet; it varies from climate to climate, season to season and sadhana to sadhana. Perhaps the ideal yogic diet can be summed up as the most natural, simplest to purchase, to prepare and digest.

Changing with the Seasons

The ancient yogic scriptures have given us extensive advice on how to maintain a sattvic diet. The recommendations vary with climate, season and personality type.

Climate – Whatever foods nature provides will allow us to adapt best to that climate. For example, in the tropics more cooling light foods such as fresh fruits and vegetables will be available. In the arctic there will be more heavy, heat producing foods – plenty of animal products and fats. Tropical foods, if consumed in the arctic, may even act as a poison as they contain the elements which the body requires for coping with extreme heat. Similarly, if large amounts of animal fats are consumed in the tropics, the digestive system will surely give trouble as the body does not require them or know how to utilize them.

In hot climates, grains and legumes are used as the staple food to provide sufficient protein and carbohydrate, then fruits and vegetables are added to complete the nutritional requirements. In cold climates, however, many people find it difficult to eat grains and lentils in a sufficient quantity to supply all their protein needs. They usually fool a need for something heavier, which can be met by taking more dairy products, eggs and nuts.

Season – During summer certain foods may make the body too hot, but if used in winter, these same foods may maintain the body heat at Just the right level. In the summer heat, the digestive fire is low and a light diet is needed. Cold weather fans the digestive fire, increasing the food requirement and allowing heavier foods to be digested.

Personality type also governs dietary needs, for example a hot tempered person should take more cooling foods and avoid those which increase heat and passion.

The ayurvedic texts give extensive advice for maintaining a sattvic diet based on the Indian climate, the 6 divisions of the year and the foods available in India.

1. *Hemant* (winter - 15th November to 15th January) : Kapha (phlegm) is aggravated by cold and the following are recommended sour, fat and salt sauces, milk preparations, sweets, fats, oils, new rice and hot liquids.

2. *Shisira* (season of dew - 15th January to 15th March) : Vata (wind) is aggravated and one should avoid pungent, cold food and drink.

3. *Vasanta* (spring - 15th March to 15th May) : Accumulated kapha can provoke many diseases and this can be remedied by emetics (such as Kunjal) and the avoidance of heavy, sour, oily and sweet food. Barley and wheat are recommended.

4. *Grishma* (summer - 15th May to 15th July) : Pitta (bile) predominates and one is advised to take tasty, cold, fluid, oily things. Avoid salt, sour, pungent and hot foods.

5. *Varsha* (rainy season - 15th July to 15th September) : Vata predominates and the digestion is particularly weak. Barley, wheat, and fermented rice, boiled sauce, honey, rain water or boiled water are recommended.

6. *Sharad* (autumn - 15th September to 15th November) : Pitta predominates and one should eat a moderate quantity of sweet, light, cold foods. Rice, barley and wheat should be taken. Pure water should be obtained from a well or spring. Bitter foods and drinks, ghee, fat and oil should be avoided.

7

Conclusion

In the course of our brief survey we have skirted many profound and important issues, all of which have a bearing, whether we realize it or not, on the relatively simply decision to stop eating meat. Readers who wish to follow up some or all of the topics touched on in this book will find a number of suggestions for further study in the Reading List. It is important for vegetarians to be informed if they are to hold their own in a still predominantly carnivorous society, and if they are to stand any change of persuading others that their dietary choice is both ethically and practically necessary.

How far, though, can one legitimately go in persuading other people to give up meat?

The hard-line approach is to assert that food habits cannot be left to personal whim or habit or the vagaries of market forces; that dietary good sense must be in some way to other, be made to prevail; that in a word' the right to eat what one please is the flesh of defenseless fellow creatures, is not an absolute one and if persisted in demands militant opposition at every opportunity.

A more moderate approach is to assume that by and large it is people's ignorance that enforces the meat habit and that it is this that is the main stumbling block to a wider extension of vegetarianism. If people knew more about the realities of modern meat production, the argument might run, and then they would make the right choices of their own volition.

This is the essence of what we called in the first edition of this book the subversive way: to place the right sort of information courteously but with firm persistence before people, whenever we have the opportunity in order to try and make them look at their traditional assumptions about what they eat in a new way.

Persuading your friends and neighbours to give up meat, it might be said, brings its own moral dilemma: is it ethical to force people into doing something that they don't want to do? It is, after all a conflict of freedoms: the freedom of certain types of animals to live out their allotted span without being slaughtered for food by human beings and the freedom of the human animal to eat what pleases him. For anyone who has considered the issues, even on a superficial level, the dilemma is a spurious one. There can be no question about it: the moral right of any creature to life—leaving aside for the moment all other consideration—it infinitely greater than the right of another creature to condemn it to live only for slaughter simply to gratify a perverted palate.

It is clear that people are changing their attitudes towards meat. At the time of writing there may be as many as 20 million people in the UK who have reduced their meat consumption over the past fifteen years and the trend towards an avoidance of meat and outright vegetarianism is now of statistical significance. The meat trade certainly thinks so and is desperately trying to share up its crumbling defences against the formidable logic of vegetarianism. Back in May 1977 the *Meat Trades journal* was pointing to the kind of association meat producers do not want their customers to make: 'to acquaint the customer' it says, 'with the knowledge that the lamb' chops she has just purchased were part of the anatomy of one of those pretty little creatures we see gamboling in the fields at springtime is probably the surest way of turning her into a vegetarian. Though we may marvel at the cynicism, the reasoning is impeccable.

Vegetarianism is not a weak-minded fad, a mere pose or a cozily sentimental feeling for animals. On the contrary, it is, or should be, a lifelong commitment, a lifestyle anchored on firm moral and intellectual convictions, a responsible acknowledgement that our species, for all its wonderful and unique gift, is only one of many with no absolute right to dispose of non-human animals and the environments in which they live merely in order to satisfy a culinary whim. That whim has already been the death of countless millions of animals, and indirectly of many human beings. It is time we grew up. There are signs that we are beginning to do so.

Bibliography

Sussman, *Vegetarian Alternative.*

Gary Null, *Protein for Vegetarians* (1975).

Akers, *Vegetarian Sourcebook.*

R.D. Bragen, *The Vegetarian's Self-Defence Manual* (1979).

John A. Scharffenberg, *Problems with Meat.*

Michael J. Hill, 'Bacteria and the Aetiology of Cancer of the Large Bowel', *The Lancet* (1971).

R.L. Phillips et at, 'Coronary Heart Disease Mortality among Seventh-day Adventists......', *American Journal of Clinical Nutrition* (1978).

Scharffenberg, *op.cit.*

R.L. Phillips, 'Role of Lifestyle and Dietary Habits in Risk of Cancer among Seventh-day Adventists,' *Cancer Research* (November 1975).

Jon Wynne-Tyson, *Food for a Future.*

Peter Burwash and John Tullio, *Peter Burwash's Vegetarian Primer.*

Akers, *Vegetarian Handbook.*

Compassion in World Farming leaflet, 'Factory Farm '79. What you can do.'

The New Vegetarian, February 1978.

Keith Akers, *A Vegetarian Sourcebook* (1983).

Nathaniel Altman, *Eating For Life* (1973).

Animal Welfare in Poutry, Pig and Veal Calf Production (HMSO, 1981).

Janet Barkas, *The Vegetable Passion* (1975).

Louis Berman, *Vegetarianism and the Fewish Tradition* (1982).

Brigid Brophy, 'The Rights of Animal' *(Sunday Times/*Vegetarian Society, 1965).

Peter Burwash and John Tullius, *Peter Burwash's Vegetarian Primer* (1983).

Stephen R.L. Clark, *The Moral Status of Animals* (1977).

— The Nature of the Beast : *Are Animals Moral?* (1982).

Marian Stamp Dawkins, *Animal Suffering* (1980).

Daniel Dombrowski, *Vegetarianism : The Philosophy Behind The Ethical Diet* (1985).

Rodger Doyle, *The Vegetarian Handbook* (1980).

Michael W. Fox, *Returning to Eden* : *Animal Rights and human Responsibility* (1980).

Dudley Giehl, *Vegetarianism : A Way of Life* (1981).

Stanley nd Roslind Godlovitch and John Harris (eds.), *Animals, Men and Morals : An Enquiry into the Mal-treatment of Non-Humans* (1972).

Donal Griffin, *The Question of Animal Awareness* (1976).

Maurice Hanssen, *E for Additives* (1984).

Ruth Harrison, *Animal Machines* (1964).

Clive Hollands, *Compassion is the Bugler* (1981).

Andrew Linzey, *Animal Rights* : *A Christian Assesement of Man's Treatment of Animals* (1976).

Charles Magel, *A Bibliography on Animal Rights and Related Matters* (1981).

Jim Mason and Peter Singer, *Animal Factories* (1980).

Mary Midgley, *Animals and Why They Matter : A Journey Round the Species Barrier* (1984).

Victoria Moran, *Compassion : The Ultimate Ethic* (1985).

R. K. Morris and M.W. Fox (eds.), *On the Fifth Day : Animal Rights and Human Ethics* (1978).

Richard North, *The Animals Report* (1984).

David Paterson and Richard D. Ryder (eds.), *Animal Rights : A Symposium* (1979).

Tom Regan, *All That Dwells Therein* (1982).

—The Case for Animal Rights (1983).

Tom Regan and Peter Singer (eds.), *Animal Rights and Human Obligations* (1976).

Report of the Technical Committeee to Enquire into the Welfare of Animals kept Under Intensive Livestock Husbandry Systems (The Brambell Report) (HMSO, 1965).

Richard Ryder, *Victims of Science* (1975).

Henry S. Salt, *Animals' Rights* (1882).

John A. Scharffenberg, *Problems With Meat* (1979).

Peter Singer, *Animal Liberation : Towards an End to Man's Inhumanity to Animals* (1976, 1983).

Vic Sussman, *The Vegetarian Alternative* (1978).

E.S. Turner, *All Heaven in a Rage* (1964).

Esme Wynne -Tyson, *The Philosophy of Compassion* (1970).

Jon Wynne-Tyson, *The Civilized Alternative* (1972).

—, *Food for a Future* (1975, 1979).

www.vegsoc.org

www.ivu.org

http://purifymind.com/BriefHisVege.htm

www.all-creatures.org/mhvs

www.vivavegie.org/vv101/vv101reas.html

http://cardiology.jwatch.org/cgi/content/full/2005/603/1

Index

E

F

G

H

M

N

O

P

R